THE TRUTH ABOUT
MELASMA

What You Need to Know About the
Root Causes of Melasma and
How to Treat It Holistically

JANETT JUWIEN

FOR MY GREATEST LOVES

MAXIMILLIAN & OZIRIS

Published by Ecvilibria
© 2022 J. Juwien
All rights reserved

Contact
Janett Juwien
janett@ecvilibria.com
ecvilibria.com

Editor Jacqueline Bain & Sophie Elletson
Designer Collette Sadler & Alex Dickson
Illustrations Collette Sadler & Janett Juwien

Paperback ISBN 9780645712001
eBook ISBN 9780645712018

CONTENTS

PREFACE

HOW THIS BOOK CAME TO BE

After working as an aesthetician for many years, I noticed that clients with melasma have risen to an alarming number. To my own and my clients' frustration, I had to tolerate the fact that professional treatments and cosmetics do not give the desired results. The information I have gathered from my clients' personal melasma stories revealed to me that this is more than just sun-induced or pregnancy-related hyperpigmentation. I decided to start the search on the medical database for answers and felt a responsibility to pass on the findings. That is where my idea for this book came to life. The aspiration with my work is to build an educational bridge regarding skin health between clinical research and the patient. I have a passion for sharing my knowledge about skin health and overall well-being with out-of-the-box thinking. I hope with all my heart that this book will help you on your healing journey from melasma.

INTRODUCTION

WHAT YOU CAN EXPECT FROM THIS BOOK

The best way to describe *The Truth About Melasma* is to categorise it as a skincare book. However, only a tiny fraction is dedicated to traditional skincare, which is the application of cosmetics. The reason is that true skincare requires the nurture of the whole body. As the book title indicates, you can expect some unveiling of the true nature of melasma.

The root cause of all skin conditions, including melasma, is an imbalance in the body caused by either toxicity, deficiency or both. Any disruption to our bodies causes an imbalance within our delicate internal environment. The result is a dysregulated nervous and endocrine system, as well as inflammation. The skin displays imbalances with redness, eruptions, brown spots and premature ageing. The simple truth is, the healthier you are, in body, mind and spirit, the more blemish free your skin looks.

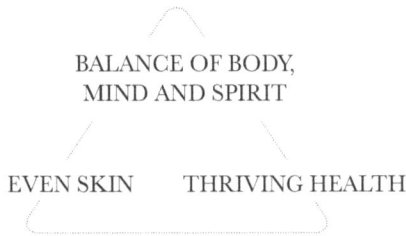

BALANCE OF BODY,
MIND AND SPIRIT

EVEN SKIN   THRIVING HEALTH

Image 1: The triangle is the most stable shape in geometry and symbolises here the stability of health when the body is in harmony (equilibrium) (Credit: Collette Sadler).

As mentioned before, this book is not a skincare book that focuses on a daily regime with instructions on how to apply creams and masks. Instead, the book will educate you about the real issues that cause melasma. It offers holistic solutions to regain homeostasis in your body so that your skin can heal and your hyperpigmentation fade. The word homeostasis is synonymous with balance of the body, e.g.. ideal body temperature, ideal water-salt balance, optimum oxygenation, balanced blood sugar, a balanced free radical and antioxidant ratio and the absence of inflammation. There truly is no alternative other than the holistic way (holistic=whole, interdependence between parts) because to heal your skin, you need to recover your entire body. To heal your body, you need to live in symbiosis and love with your mind, body, spirit and your environment. The skin is the barrier between the outer and inner environment and therefore not only responds to the environment but also reflects what is going on in your inner and outer world simultaneously.

The book is divided into four Parts. Part I conveys general facts about melasma. Part II follows with the presentation of the clinical evidence that shows how imbalances in the body are correlated to melasma. Part III suggests factors that cause these imbalances, while Part IV offers holistic solutions.

PART I.

GENERAL FACTS ABOUT MELASMA

MELASMA AT A GLANCE

Melasma is a skin hyperpigmentation that appears mainly on the face. Other areas of the body can be affected, but the expression of melasma on the face is the most common. Dark, large and symmetrically organised patches are typical features, as seen in the image below.

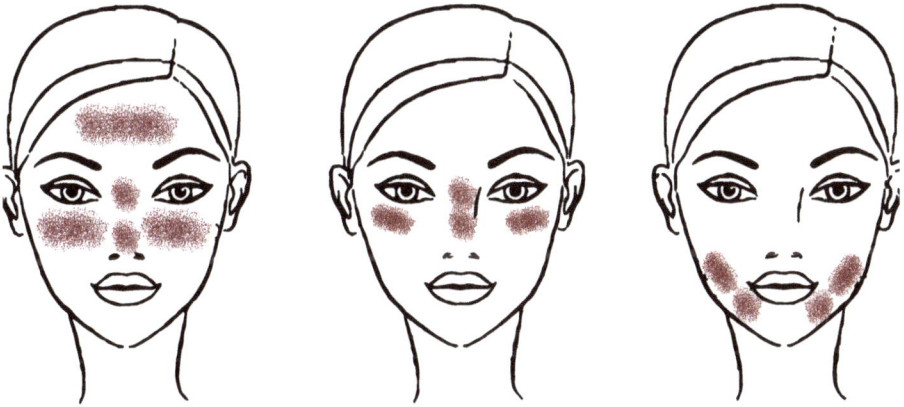

Image 2: A typical presentation of melasma.

THE COMMON BELIEF
Melasma is caused by raised estrogen levels and sun exposure.

THE FACTS
Many women who suffer from melasma have not been pregnant or taken contraceptive pills.

Men can have melasma [1].

Melasma does not fade despite the use of sunblock or the avoidance of sunlight.

Melasma is more common in darker skin types that should innately be more protected against sun damage.

The research on melasma and skin hyperpigmentation points to imbalances in the nervous and endocrine systems, inflammation and oxidative stress. Those imbalances are the result of toxicities, deficiencies or both. Because all of our body systems are connected, we must maintain and regain balance in our whole body by removing the toxicity and restoring the deficiencies as efficiently as possible.

TOXICITY/OVERLOAD	DEFICIENCY
Stress	Vitamin D
Copper → causes high estrogen	Nutrients
Air pollution	Oxygen → increase of blood vessel formation
Gut bacteria	Gut bacteria
Endocrine disruptors	Antioxidants → causing oxidative stress
Chemicals	
Artificial light	
Medications	
Metals	
UV radiation	

Table 1: Toxicities and deficiencies that cause imbalances.

HYPERPIGMENTATION EXPLAINED SIMPLY

Before we learn about melasma in more detail, let's lay the foundation and have a quick dip into hyperpigmentation.

Hyperpigmentation of the skin is characterised by an overly dark colouring of certain areas due to the increase of the pigment melanin. Melanin is the pigment that the body produces to give our hair, eyes and skin their typical tone. In the skin, this pigment is produced by melanocytes in the epidermis (Image 3). There are different components that are needed to build melanin, which are the amino acid tyrosine, an enzyme called tyrosinase, oxygen and sunlight.

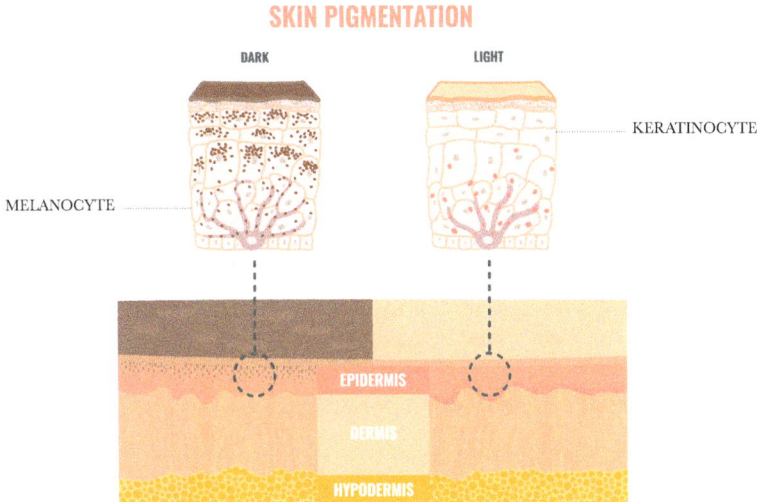

Image 3: A classic skin diagram (Credit: art4stock).

Melanin production is a mechanism of the skin to protect itself from harmful environmental factors, such as Ultraviolet Radiation (UVR) from the atmosphere. UV radiation is part of the natural sunlight. The warming and nurturing rays of the sun we all love are essential for our health and well-being, but the highly energetic charge of ultraviolet rays can be harmful if we are overly exposed. UVR is considered harmful because of the damage it can do to the DNA in the cell core. Melanin, produced by cells called melanocytes, protects the skin from the sun by absorbing UV radiation. As nature has designed all species to survive and reproduce, the body will always prioritise the protection of DNA. Whenever the DNA is in danger, defence responses are activated.

The immune system is the defence mechanism that reacts to sunburn after too much sun exposure. Sometimes the sunburn turns into a tan; sometimes, the damage is so extensive that skin cells die and shed (peeling effect). When the DNA gets damaged, but the cell does not die, the cell divides with flawed genetic information, resulting in cancer.

Melanin has a staggering role as a neutraliser for radiation, free radicals, and chemicals [2]. It can be considered an antioxidant that acts whenever skin cells require protection. The darker the skin is, the more melanin it contains, meaning more UV rays and stressors can be absorbed, thereby reducing cell destruction. After melanin is produced by melanocytes, it is then transferred to the surrounding keratinocytes. All of these cells are located in the epidermis (Image 3).

Healthy pigmentation, also called tan, is a natural progression and shows up as an even colour on the skin in different shades of brown, depending on your skin type (Fitzpatrick scale Table 2). The skin type is determined by genetics due to heritage and geographical location of origin but can be influenced by environmental factors such as sun exposure.

	I	II	III	IV	V	VI
HERITAGE	North European/ Irish	North European/ Swedish	Mediter-ranean	East Asian/ Indian	Indian/ South American/ African	African
HAIR	Red Blond	Blond Red Dark Blond	Chestnut Dark Blond	Brown/ Medium Brown/ Dark Brown	Dark Brown	Black
EYES	Blue Grey Green	Blue Grey Green Hazel	Brown Blue Grey Green Hazel	Brown	Brown	Brown
SKIN	Pale Freckles	Pale	Pale/ Light Brown	Medium Brown/ Dark Brown	Dark Brown	Dark Brown/ Black

Table 2: Skin type scale after Fitzpatrick.

The even tan is an "orderly" state of hyperpigmentation achieved under the most common circumstance, which is sun exposure. Sun exposure or UV radiation is the most common external factor to influence the intensity of pigmentation. Internal factors that stimulate pigmentation are hormones, such as estrogen. Those internal and external circumstances lead to morphological changes in melanocytes, which result in uneven skin colour. We will discuss all these circumstances in Part II and III.

When uneven pigmentation shows as freckles, age spots, moles or larger patches, certain characteristics show when the skin is viewed under the microscope. These are:

1. An increased number of melanocytes.

2. Melanocytes contain more melanin.

3. Melanocytes are enlarged.

4. Their dendrites (arms) are longer and more abundant.

5. Another typical feature is the increased activity of the enzyme tyrosinase (not visible under the microscope).

These characteristics can occur simultaneously.

FACTS ABOUT MELASMA

Melasma is a form of hyperpigmentation that typically displays on the face and is primarily associated with pregnancy and sun exposure. Early records documented melasma only in pregnant women, which is why it is also labelled as a "mask of pregnancy". The main contributing factor for melasma during pregnancy is an increased level of the female sex hormone estrogen and placental hormones. Women on "the pill" (birth control contraception) often develop melasma, which reinforces the belief that estrogen is to blame. However, melasma also affects women who have no history of pregnancy or taking the pill; it affects men [1] and the transgender population [3].

The sun, often blamed and therefore shunned, is the other main factor believed to cause melasma. This is not an entirely wrong assumption since the sun is known to form the most common type of hyperpigmentation, the tan. But how is it possible that more and more people develop melasma while humans spend more time indoors than we have over the last hundred years? The clients I have consulted have rigorously used sunscreen daily out of fear of forming more pigmentation. The use of sunscreen had neither prevented brown patches nor led to fading. This raises the question: What factors other than oral contraceptives, pregnancy or sun exposure drive this skin condition?

Elevated estrogen levels can indeed cause hyperpigmentation, but estrogen can rise by several external factors. Some of these factors are chemicals that hide in cosmetic products. Ironically, despite the belief that sunscreen is essential for people with melasma, some UV filters act as hormone disruptors resulting in increased estrogen levels. Oxybenzone, for example, is a widely used chemical UV filter and is known to mimic estrogen.

Additionally, many sunscreens do not have equivalent UVA and UVB filters in their formula. The main concern of sunscreen developers and formulators is to prevent sunburn. Sunburn is caused by UVB light. Because the main goal is to prevent sunburn, manufacturers often focus on UVB protection. Hence the SPF claim (15, 20, 30, 50+) on the bottles often only stands for the UVB filter, not the UVA filter [4]. A broad-spectrum sunscreen will have filters for both types of UV, but the UVA filter might be lower. That means the two types of rays are split into different degrees of protection and penetration, which can aggravate pigmentation.

The pattern of melasma is significant, as it appears symmetrically and favours the cheeks, forehead, nose and upper lip area. People with naturally darker skin types are more prone to develop melasma. Regarding the skin cells, it is typical that the melanocytes are bigger and contain more melanin than usual, while their actual number is not increased. Furthermore, the hyperpigmented areas in melasma are not only found in the epidermal layer, where brown pigment should be but also underneath, the dermal layer (dermis). The fact that lesions are found in the dermis is likely a reason why melasma is harder to treat. Tattoos, for example, are purposely placed in the dermis to make them last forever.

Wood's lamps are widely used in skin therapy studios as skin diagnosis tools. When examining the skin, this lamp is a helpful tool to find out if pigmentation is present in the dermis. If the melasma lesions, or part of them, are not visible under the wood's lamp, we have dermal pigmentation. The reason is simply that the light emitted by the wood's lamp cannot reach into the deeper dermal layers. You only see what is in the epidermis.

THE HISTORY

The first descriptions of melasma can be found in the medical literature extending as far back as the reports of Hippocrates (470–360 BC). The term was used to designate a series of skin pigmentation processes. Back then, Hippocrates had already observed that melasma worsened after sun exposure, fire, heat, cold and skin inflammations [5].

TYPICAL FEATURES

1. Melasma appears in distinctive patterns and a symmetrical fashion.

2. Increased activity and increased size of melanocytes [6].

3. Increased melanin content in melanocytes [6][7].

4. The number of melanocytes is not increased [7].

5. Increased tyrosinase activity.

6. Epidermal thinning with defective barrier [8].

7. Melanin can also be present in the dermis as opposed to only the epidermis [7].

8. A disrupted basement membrane. This is a situation where the barrier between the epidermis and dermis is damaged. It can allow the epidermal melanin to leak into the dermis and is one of the possible reasons why we find melasma there [9][10].

9. Increased number of blood vessels (vascularity) around melasma lesions.

10. Increased mast cell count in melasma lesions.

Scenarios 3, 6, 7, 8, 9 and 10 are depicted in the image below (Image 4).

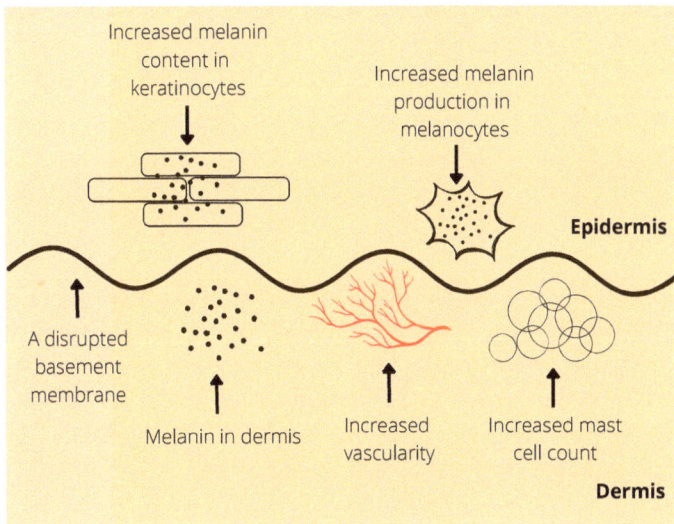

Image 4: Typical histological features of melasma.

To follow a root cause-based healing approach to melasma, we need to ask why these typical features occur. For example:

What makes melanocytes overactive?

Why is the pigmentation appearing in large patches in a distinctive pattern?

Why is melasma always showing up symmetrically?

What makes melanocytes increase in size?

What increases tyrosinase activity?

Why do we find melanin in the dermis?

Why do we have a defective barrier?

What is responsible for a thinning epidermis?

Why do we see more blood vessels around the lesions?

Why do we find mast cells in melasma lesions?

We will explore all these questions and potential answers in Part II and III.

THE DEMOGRAPHICS

If you prefer not to read about the demographics of melasma, you can skip to the next chapter. It is not essential to understand Part II or III, and you can always come back to it at a later time.

GENDER

80% female

20% male [11][1].

PHOTOTYPE

Melasma seems to be more prevalent in darker phototypes from type III and above (Fitzpatrick type). Two independent studies from Brazil conducted a survey of 300 and 950 melasma patients, respectively. 34–36% of patients had phototype III, while 38–40% had phototype VI [12][13]. It is assumed that people with darker skin have a greater potential to experience melasma, as their melanocytes are more responsive than in lighter skin types.

FAMILY HISTORY

A correlation to family history is possible, but the result ranges between 18% and 65% of four different surveys. When we speak about family history, we consider the impact of genetics. The question is: do we inherit a gene for melasma, or the gene for the skin colour, that makes us more susceptible to hyperpigmentation? Or do lifestyle habits play a more significant part? You will find a paragraph on the topic of genetics in Part II.

Family history reported between 18%–65% [12][14][15][11].

PREGNANCY

For 13.6%–27% of women, pregnancy is their onset event [11][15].

ORAL CONTRACEPTIVE

18%–38% of patients reported a correlation between beginning the oral contraceptive pill and their initial onset of melasma [11][15][16].

AGE OF ONSET

For most patients, the age of onset seems to be around 30 years [14][11].

PATTERN

Patterns in skin conditions are common and can reflect the underlying issue. Melasma appears symmetrically on the face. This consistent presentation is a good indicator for skin diagnosis. The typical, symmetrical branching in melasma can be a reflection of the peripheral nerve routes, which we will come to later in Part II, "Melasma and The Nervous System".

There are three different patterns in melasma:

1. Centrofacial

2. Malar

3. Mandibular

The table below shows where the pigmentation in the three different patterns sits.

	NOSE	UPPER CHEEKS	LOWER CHEEKS	FORE-HEAD	UPPER LIP	CHIN
CENTROFACIAL	+	+		+	+	+
MALAR	+	+				
MANDIBULAR			+			

Table 3: Location of melasma in the different patterns.

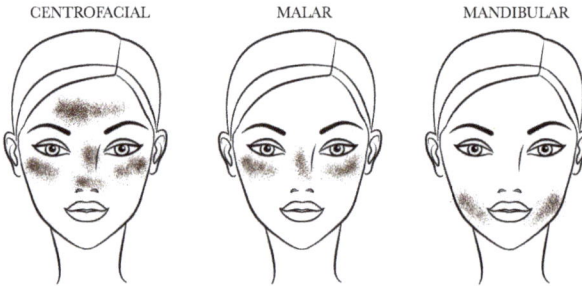

CENTROFACIAL   MALAR   MANDIBULAR

Image 5: The three different melasma patterns (Credit: Julia White & Collette Sadler).

According to the surveys, most patients will have a centrofacial or malar pattern. I have averaged the following percentages from seven sources.

Centrofacial: 29–76%

Malar: 20–71%

Mandibular: 10–15% [7][17][18][1][11][15][16]

At the end of Part II, you will learn what traditional Chinese face reading can tell you about the melasma patterns and why they display at a particular location.

EPIDERMAL AND DERMAL DISTRIBUTION

Out of 138/312 patients from two different studies had:

Epidermal melasma: 21–50%

Dermal melasma: 35–55%

Mixed (epidermal and dermal): 15–24% [18][11]

PART II

THE ROOT CAUSES OF MELASMA — HOW IMBALANCES CAUSE HYPERPIGMENTATION

INTRODUCTION TO PART II

In this chapter, we explore how the nervous, endocrine, and immune systems as well as cellular breathing are related to melasma.

The common belief is that only the female sex hormone estrogen and sun exposure are to blame for melasma. The link of melasma to estrogen is generally correct and originates from the observation that it occurs in women during pregnancy. It is still labelled colloquially as "the pregnancy mask". Since oral contraceptives ("the pill") became popular, melasma has also been reported to be a common side effect in women on the pill.

The reason is that melanocytes respond to estrogen, which subsequently activates the pigmentation process. Estrogen levels are higher in pregnant women and also increased when taking the pill. As the melanocytes become activated and overly stimulated by the excess estrogen in the body, pregnant women typically experience a darkening of the nipples and areolas and the snail trail below the belly button as a consequence of hormonal changes.

The system that controls hormones, like estrogen, is called the endocrine or hormone system. The endocrine system also regulates our stress hormones, thyroid hormones and even blood sugar.

In this chapter, I reveal how hormones other than estrogen play a role in the development of melasma and how this skin condition can be a sign of imbalances in the entire endocrine system. Also, we will find out how the nervous system and immune system are connected to the skin and how this connection affects skin pigmentation. We will also explore the impacts of oxidative stress. Let's dive in.

The skin is connected and in communication with the nervous, endocrine and immune systems. Our skin has its own immune system but is also affected when the systemic immune system of our respiratory and digestive systems is alerted. The connection between the systems stems from the origin these systems shared during our embryonic stage and their close proximity at that time. In the picture below, you see a gastrula:

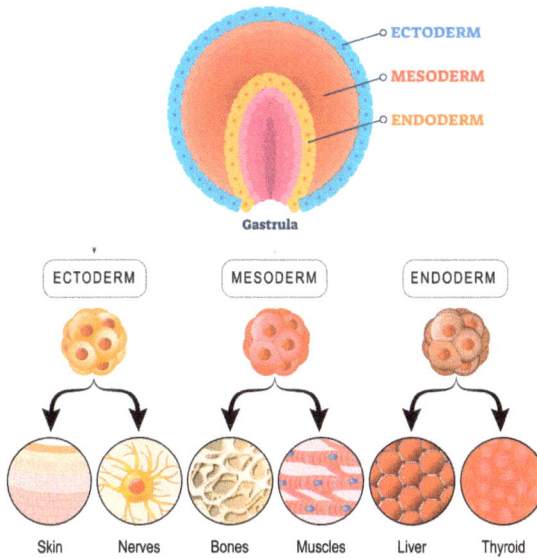

Image 6: A three weeks old embryo (Gastrula)(Credit: by VectorMine & ttsz).

The gastrula, depicted in the image above, was you when you were three weeks old; only a little ball made up of cells in three differentiated layers. The fate of each layer was already predetermined. The outer layer would later become the nervous system and the skin; the middle layer becomes muscles, skeleton, kidneys and reproductive organs and the inner layer other endocrine glands, lungs, digestive organs and liver. In the course of maturation and growth, to the time when we are fully developed, and until we die, all of these body parts will stay connected through a complex highway of pathways.

The endocrine, nervous and immune systems interact with each other to keep homeostasis (balance) in your body and ensure survival and repair. The interaction between these three systems happens on the systemic level but also between the local nervous, endocrine and immune systems of the skin. Furthermore, the systemic systems respond to the local systems and vice versa [19]. It is certainly not easy to comprehend this enormous highway in the body, but the complexity of it also demonstrates the approach we need to take to treat skin conditions, as the skin is not an isolated organ.

When the systems are overstimulated or not functioning properly due to stressors, the body is out of balance, and we get sick. The skin is the organ that often shows these imbalances. Long before we feel pain or have serious problems, the skin responds with rashes, itchiness, inflammation, and other irregularities. It is the window to the body, and the body uses the skin as a communication medium. The skin has the role of ensuring homeostasis within the body and is the barrier between the outer and inner environment.

Any stressor perceived or absorbed by the skin can disrupt systemic and local homeostasis. In case of disruptions, the systemic and local systems are activated as defence and repair mechanisms to enact healing. Stress that is perceived and processed by the immune, nervous and endocrine systems, often evokes a reaction that can be seen on the skin. For example, psychological states like anxiety, fear, shame, pleasure, and sexual excitation are visibly indicated by blushing, hair-rising, growing pale, itching or sweating. The skin undoubtedly responds to many psychological and stressful stimuli [20]. Why is that important for us? Suppose the skin is responding to stimuli with sensations like itch and colour like paleness or redness. Is it not possible that hyperpigmentation, such as melasma, can be a response to daily stressors? According to researchers, the skin is a stress organ, and its pigmentary activity serves as a unique sensor and translator of stressors and a regulator of homeostasis [21]. But what are those stressors?

THE EFFECTS OF STRESS ON THE SYSTEMS — WHAT ARE STRESSFUL STIMULI?

Everyone talks about stress as the villain to blame for all sorts of ailments. And when modern medicine does not have a better answer to our symptoms, it can be frustrating to hear that stress is the cause of our health condition. Don't we all experience stress? Here is an example of what stress is by definition: "Stress arises when people are under mental, physical, or emotional pressure. It arises when the individual perceives that the pressure exceeds his adaptive power. Stress is perceived by the nervous system, endocrine system and immune system. This triggers various physiological and behavioural changes and responses that try to adapt the body to the stress" [22]. Or simpler, stress is perceived when the pressure is higher than the stamina. Emotional, physical and mental pressure covers a vast spectrum. If we brainstorm and write down stressors, we could probably fill a sheet of paper the size of a football field. We discuss the stress response in depth in this chapter titled "Melasma and Stress", and we will talk more about stress factors in Part III.

EXAMPLES OF STRESSORS	
Physical	Emotional/Mental
Chemicals, toxins, metals	Traumatic events
Radiation and artificial light	Fear
Heat	Workload and responsibilities
Physical damage, pressure, injury, etc.	Losses
Free radicals	Separation

Table 4: Examples of stressors that disrupt the systems.

Our melanocytes, which hold the most meaningful position in skin pigmentation disorders, respond to and interact with the nervous, endocrine and immune systems. The connection of melasma to these systems has sparked great interest in clinical research. I will present these findings to you in the following chapters.

MELASMA AND THE NERVOUS SYSTEM

A SHORT INTRODUCTION

The nervous system is like an electrical highway made up of nerves that span your entire body. This network transports electrical messages along the nerves. It consists of the spinal cord, brain and all the nerves that extend into all tissues and organs of your body.

This system interprets information coming from the senses. The senses are the first unit that receives stress and activates the nervous system via electrical messages, also known as impulses, that travel along the nerves. The electrical processes of the nervous system and the chemical processes of the endocrine system are joined together. The nervous system can activate or calm the endocrine system.

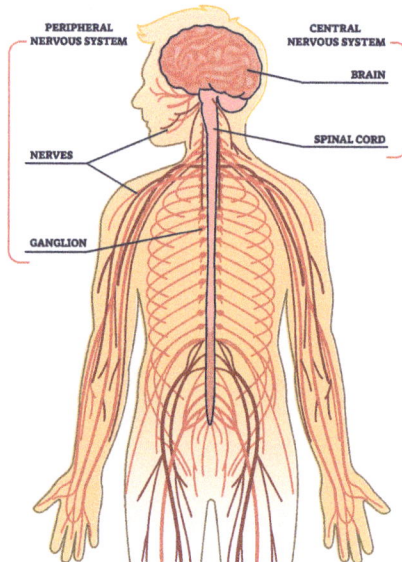

Image 7: The nervous system (Credit: VectorMine).

HOW MELANOCYTES AND THE NERVOUS SYSTEM ARE CONNECTED

Nerve cells (neurons) and melanocytes are connected due to their shared origin from the neural tube. The neural tube is the embryonic precursor to the central nervous system, which is made up of the brain and spinal cord and owned by all animal embryos with a spine, from fish to humans. Both types of cells, nerve cells and melanocytes, derive from the same stem cell lineage. After their development in the neural tube, they travel to their end destinations. The melanocytes to the skin, eyes and hair follicles and the neurons to the brain, muscles, organs, eyes, skin and other locations. After that, they will stay connected by the nervous system and specific cell signalling pathways (e.g. cAMP and Wnt pathway) and get triggered by external and internal stimuli [23]. This connection enables the skin to respond to the nervous system, which is desired in certain situations like sweating (to cool down the body).

THE LINK TO THE TRIGEMINAL NERVE

Modern science suggests a potential connection between melasma and the nervous system due to the preferred location of pigmented patches along the trigeminal nerves. Furthermore, several clinical investigations have shown that neuroactive molecules, liberated by nerve endings, have a stimulatory effect on melanocytes. Those neuroactive molecules were also present in melasma patients [24]. If we look at the image below, we see three different melasma patterns with their preferred location on the face (right side). Now comparing the location of melasma lesions to the location of the three different trigeminal nerve types (left side), we can see a striking similarity.

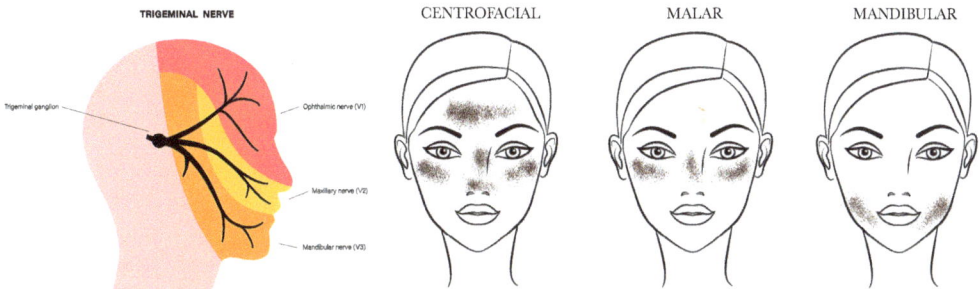

Image 8: Comparison of the melasma patterns and zones of the trigeminal nerve (Credit: Pikovit44, juliawhite & Collette Sadler).

First, a short exploration of the trigeminal nerve:

The trigeminal nerve is the largest cranial nerve and is connected to the vagus nerve (the vagus nerve is involved in the fight/flight and rest/digest response). The branches of the trigeminal nerve originate in the skin and mucosa of the face and end in the brain. Its function is to send sensory information such as pain, temperature change, touch and contact with chemicals on the facial skin, nose, mouth mucosa and eyes to the brain. The received sensory information will then trigger the release of chemicals in the brain to induce further reactions to defend or protect the body. Sensory information can be the pain you feel in your mouth when eating something very spicy or the tickle in your nose when you inhale an irritant. The typical reaction to spicy food can include tearing eyes and a tickle in the nose leading to a sneeze. Also, the burning feeling on the skin when you have applied something irritating is the sensory work of the trigeminal nerve.

The trigeminal nerve is also involved in muscle movement and transfers motor information to chewing muscles. The response to chemicals by the trigeminal nerve is called chemoreception and is typically activated by chemicals classified as irritants, including air pollutants. Air pollutants can be carbon dioxide and diesel particles from fuel combustion. Some chemical irritants can be highly concentrated alcohol or hot spices, for example [25].

Circling back to the study that has looked at the connection between melasma and the nervous system. The research team obtained skin samples of six women from lesional and non-lesional skin to compare the receptor expression of the neuroactive molecule nerve growth factor (NGF) and neural endopeptidase (NEP) (both involved in trigeminal nerve activity). They found that the keratinocytes of melasma lesions had an increased sensitivity to NGF, increased NEP and that pigmented areas were more innervated by trigeminal nerve endings [24]. So, what does it mean for us?

THE NERVE GROWTH FACTOR—HOW MELASMA IS LINKED TO EMOTIONAL STATES AND ENVIRONMENTAL TOXINS

NGF is a molecule that ensures the growth of nerve tissue, which is generally essential for the survival, development and maintenance of neurons. NEP is an enzyme that helps the breakdown of NGF. Therefore, an increased level of NEP indicates an increased level of NGF. In vitro studies demonstrated the growth of new nerve fibres after the incubation of tissue with NGF [26]. NGF is also believed to have a modulatory role in maintaining stable conditions (homeostasis) in the interaction between the nervous, endocrine and immune system (neuro-immuno-endocrine function).

Elevated NGF levels were observed in patients with autoimmune conditions, such as lupus and are generally involved in health conditions with tissue inflammation [27][28]. A study noted significantly higher NGF levels in 49 patients with chronic inflammatory disorders, asthma and allergies (food and pollen) compared to healthy controls. The patients with allergies to food and pollen had the highest levels of NGF [29][30].

The research shows that the presence of NGF and inflammation in tissues are correlated. Since NGF is released by nerve endings, the inflammation seems to be fired by the nervous system. It is long known that inflammatory states of the nervous system can manifest in skin disorders, such as atopic dermatitis. Because NGF is observed in melasma lesions, it seems this skin disorder is an inflammatory condition induced by the nervous system.

NGF is typically released by nerve endings but is also liberated by fibroblasts in the dermis and keratinocytes in the epidermis [31]. It aids in wound healing of the skin when there is inflammation [32]. Therefore, we can conclude that NGF release from skin cells is an inflammatory response, possibly after injury or contact with irritants.

Melanocytes possess NGF receptors, enabling them to respond to NGF released by fibroblasts. The response forms new dendrites [31], which means that melanin can reach more keratinocytes to turn them brown. A research team demonstrated that NGF was secreted by fibroblasts from melasma lesions and is likely responsible for the increased activity of melanocytes with the consequence of hyperpigmentation [33]. This explains how hyperpigmentation can be induced by the nervous system and also indicates that damage to the fibroblasts and inflammation in the dermis is involved in melasma.

The reason for higher NGF levels and trigeminal nerve activity is environmental factors, such as air pollution. As an example, a study shows that air pollution triggers the NGF release in rats. Researchers exposed their study subjects to diesel exhaust particles for 14 days. They found an increased level of NGF and airway inflammation [34]. Another study on rats demonstrated that inhaled ozone (O_3) induced the rise of NGF in airways [35]. Ozone naturally occurs in the atmosphere but is also generated from vehicle exhaust particles and industrial smog. The damaging effects of air pollution on our nervous system and the inflammatory repercussions are intensively researched. Is it possible that melasma is a skin condition caused by a neuronal-driven inflammatory state induced by toxins in our air?

Research suggests that the release of NGF is also linked to emotional stress as it helps the regulation of physiological homeostasis and behavioural coping. Several studies on mice and humans have proven that the release of NGF is directly related to stressful events (labour, lactation and parachute jumping) [36] [37]. In 1994, a research team investigated the effects of emotional stress on NGF in soldiers before and after their first parachute jump. The soldier's NGF levels rose to over 80 % right before the jump and more than 100 % shortly after the jump [38]. Another trial that researched emotional states reported increased NGF levels in lactating mice accompanied by aggressive behaviour [39]. We do not have clinical reports regarding NGF levels in lactating women. Still, I remember two clients who disclosed that their melasma appeared during the breastfeeding period (but not during their pregnancies).

SUMMARY—MELASMA AND THE NERVOUS SYSTEM

Let us review the facts we have covered thus far:

Nervous System

- Neuroactive molecules, such as NGF, are found in melasma.

- NGF promotes melanin production.

- Melasma is prevalent alongside trigeminal nerve branches.

Skin cells, including melanocytes, are directly connected to the nervous system. Melasma appears along the trigeminal nerve. Neuroactive molecules released by the trigeminal nerve are present in pigmented lesions and were demonstrated to evoke an increased dendricity of melanocytes. We found that NGF is linked to air pollution, respiratory and autoimmune conditions, inflammation and emotional stress. We do not know the exact reason why we find NGF in melasma lesions and still have to discover the link between the trigeminal nerve and melasma.

Nevertheless, the evidence points to a link between melasma and triggers like exhaust, emotional traumatic events and allergens that cause inflammation. There is a lot more evidence coming later on the connection between inflammation and melasma in the chapters "Melasma and the Immune System" and "Melasma and Oxidative Stress" in Part II, as well as in "Air Pollution" in Part III. You will also find more about the connection to emotional stress in the following text and I will provide you with solutions in Part IV.

MELASMA AND THE ENDOCRINE SYSTEM

AN INTRODUCTION

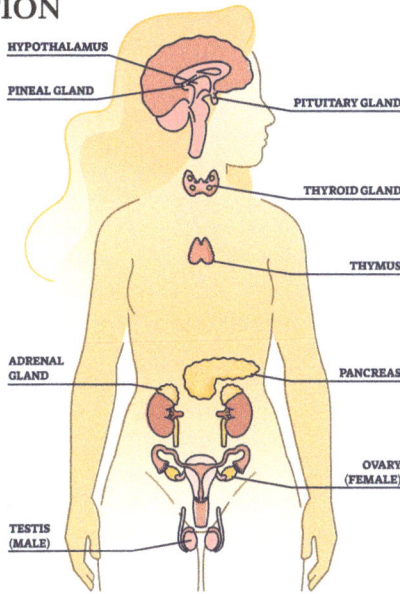

Image 9: The glands of the endocrine system (Credit: VectorMine).

The endocrine system is made up of glands that produce and secrete hormones to regulate important functions in the body including metabolism and sexual function. Hormones are chemical messengers that float in your bloodstream and transfer information from one set of cells to another to coordinate functions between different parts of the body.

In the following text, I will give you insight into the connection between the different endocrine glands (pituitary, thyroid, adrenal glands and ovaries) and melasma. Many skin problems are a reflection of imbalances in the hormone system. This is common knowledge about acne, for example. If we understand why the endocrine system becomes disrupted, we can understand the development of melasma better and find satisfying long-term solutions.

THE MAJOR GLANDS OF THE ENDOCRINE SYSTEM AND THEIR FUNCTION

HYPOTHALAMUS

The hypothalamus is the starter gland of the endocrine system and sits in the centre of your brain. The activity and release of hormones of all other glands in the endocrine system are dependent on the start signal from the hypothalamus. The major function of the hypothalamus is maintaining homeostasis in the body by responding appropriately when receiving internal and external stimuli.

INTERNAL STIMULI	EXTERNAL STIMULI
Blood pressure	Light
Blood osmolarity—Hydration	Pain
Blood sugar levels	Temperature

Table 5: Stimuli of the hypothalamus.

PINEAL GLAND

Secretion of:

- Serotonin

- Melatonin—melatonin is one of the most potent antioxidants produced in the body [40].

PITUITARY GLAND—"MASTER GLAND"

Front part (anterior) secretion of:

- Thyroid stimulating hormone (TSH)—makes T3 and T4 in your thyroid

- Adrenocorticotropin (ACTH)—makes cortisol in your adrenals

- Follicle stimulating hormone (FSH)—makes estrogen in your ovaries

- Luteinizing hormone (LH)—for ovulation in your ovaries

- Prolactin —for breast milk production

- Growth hormone—for well-being, muscle and bone health, fat metabolism

Back part (posterior) secretion of:

- Antidiuretic hormone ADH (vasopressin)—to regulate hydration

- Oxytocin—for bonding in breastfeeding, bonding after sex, often referred to as the "cuddle hormone"

THYROID

Secretion of:

- Triiodothyronine (T3)

- Thyroxine (T4)

- Keeps the body's homeostasis

- Regulates body temperature

- Regulates metabolism

PARATHYROID

- Senses calcium levels in blood via parathyroid hormone (PTH) for the proper function of muscles, bones and nerves.

ADRENALS

Secretion of:

- Cortisol

- Adrenaline

- Regulation of metabolism

- Immune system and blood pressure

PANCREAS

Secretion of:

- Insulin—rises after eating when blood serum levels of glucose rise, glucose for cellular breathing

- Digestive enzymes to break down food, e.g., lipase

OVARIES (AND TESTES):

Secretion of sex hormones (sex hormone production is affected by sunlight and melatonin levels):

- Estrogen

- Progesterone

- Testosterone

HOW ESTROGEN IS MADE IN THE BODY

When light enters the eyes, the absorbed light energy is converted into electrical energy and stimulates the secretion of gonadotropin releasing hormone (GnRH) in the preoptic area of the hypothalamus in a pulsating fashion (eyes and hypothalamus are connected). GnRH stimulates the release of FSH (follicle stimulating hormone) and LH (luteinising hormone) in the pituitary gland. From there, FSH and LH stimulate the excretion of estrogen, progesterone and testosterone in the ovaries every few hours, depending on where the menstrual cycle is at that stage. Estrogen can also be produced by fat tissue and the adrenal glands after menopause, which is meaningful for people with excess weight and continuing stress.

More recent research accepts the gut, skin and even the heart as parts of the endocrine system. With more and more research we realise that we only challenge ourselves when we try to see organs and systems as separate entities. It is now known that the gut microbiome metabolise sex hormones [41][42], the skin produces and responds to stress and sex hormones [19][21] and the ability of the heart to move blood is regulated by hormones that are produced in heart cells [43][44].

WHAT IS THE JOB OF THE ENDOCRINE SYSTEM?

The job of the endocrine system is to keep homeostasis (balance) within your body. Imbalances in the endocrine system can lead to disorders of any organ or gland involved in this system. We know that melanocytes communicate with the glands of the endocrine system and that imbalances lead to disorders of melanocytes. The proper interaction between your nervous system and the endocrine system must be ensured for the body to respond appropriately to environmental stimuli. Any inappropriate response of these two systems would over-activate the immune system and can lead to acute and chronic inflammation.

The endocrine system responds to internal and external stimuli. One example of an external stimulus is light, while an appropriate response to light would be the scenario of hormone synthesis. In the case of estrogen synthesis, light enters the eye and stimulates the hypothalamus, which further sets off a cascade of reactions in the pituitary gland and eventually the ovaries (you can find a more thorough description in "How Estrogen is Made in the Body").

An internal stimulus, for example, is the salt and water ratio of your cells (osmolarity/hydration). If your salt and water ratio is off balance, you feel sick because your endocrine system gets disrupted, which can manifest as symptoms like headaches, for example. That is why you have a hangover after a big night. You have thrown off your salt and water ratio because of intaking too much alcohol, which is why it feels so good to drink water and eat salty food, as it gets the water-salt ratio back into balance.

The body is always geared towards balance (homeostasis) and the job of the endocrine system is to do exactly that for your body and your skin. The endocrine system works on a systemic and local level. The systemic reaction refers to the whole body while hormones are floating through your blood vessels and the local system works on the spot at a particular location. The systemic and local systems interact with each other. Both can send messages to each other to maintain balance.

THE FEEDBACK LOOP—HOW THE SYSTEM NATURALLY REGULATES HORMONE RELEASE

Our endocrine system provides us with hormones to regulate body functions when exposed to stimuli like external or internal stressors. Luckily this system is smart and is able to stop the hormone production itself once the stimulus is gone and everything is back to normal levels (homeostasis). This happens due to a process called a feedback loop (there is a positive and a negative feedback loop).

Example of a negative feedback loop—estrogen production:

Your ovaries start releasing estrogen when they have received the signal (FSH and LH release) from the pituitary gland. Once the ovaries have released enough estrogen, the stimulating hormones in the hypothalamus and pituitary stop sending out FSH and LH, to stop your ovaries from producing estrogen [45]. This feedback loop applies to all endocrine glands, your thyroid, adrenals, pancreas, ovaries and testicles for males. The negative feedback loop keeps the hormone in balance through stimulation and repression mechanisms, but it can become dysregulated due to reasons we will discuss in Part III. The effects of the dysregulation can make you feel off-kilter, and if ignored, more severe damage and chronic illness can develop over time.

Note: Estrogen production in women also undergoes a positive feedback loop before ovulation but to keep this simple, I have only described the negative feedback loop in this example.

Example of a positive feedback loop—breastfeeding

When a baby sucks on the mother's nipple, the sensory nerves send impulses that stimulate the prolactin production in the pituitary gland, which leads to more milk production, until the milk is used up. In this scenario, milk production stimulates the prolactin release and the hormone release encourages milk production.

RECEPTORS: THE KEY AND LOCK SYSTEM—HOW CELLS RESPOND TO HORMONES

Another important aspect in understanding the hormone system is the receptor function, which I call the key and lock system. Receptors are protein fragments that sit on top or inside your cell and wait for the hormone to attach to them, so they can stimulate the cell to turn on its particular function. This is like a key and lock system. You can only open the door if you have the key (hormone) to fit into the lock (receptor). One of the reasons the endocrine system can get dysregulated is that these receptors can get confused. And one of the factors that can lead to confused receptors is a specific group of chemicals that are called "endocrine disruptors". These disruptors are chemicals found in cosmetics, heavy metals, household products and fungi.

Endocrine disruptors are able to mimic a hormone (acting as a fake estrogen) and dock onto the estrogen receptor. Although it is only a mimic hormone, it makes the gland believe it needs to send out more hormones. This is because the other glands do not get the message from the cell that it has received enough of the hormone to stop production because the receptor is simply blocked. This makes the gland overactive, which not only results in inflammation and exhaustion of the gland but also an overproduction and oversecretion of hormones. These blocked hormone receptors can lead to consistently elevated estrogen levels. We know that excess estrogen can be a contributing reason to the development of melasma. If the cell receptors are blocked by a fake hormone, the ovaries believe they have to release more hormones, and they will continue to do so to no end. And unfortunately, melasma is not the worst-case scenario of this. Even more alarming is the risk of breast cancer and endometrial cancer due to the effects of prolonged increased estrogen levels. We will discuss endocrine disruptors in Part III.

Autoimmune conditions can also cause hormone imbalances. Usually, the immune system sends out antibodies to target invaders. When you have an autoimmune disorder, your body sends out antibodies constantly and these antibodies can mimic hormones. One example is TSH receptor autoantibodies (TRAb) that may either mimic the action of TSH and cause the thyroid to overstimulate, or alternatively, antagonize the action of TSH and cause the thyroid to under function (hypothyroidism). The overstimulation as the result of antibody action is seen in Graves's disease which has skin hyperpigmentation as a common symptom [46].

Below are some typical symptoms of endocrine imbalances:

IMBALANCE IN:	SYMPTOM OF IMBALANCE:
Hypothalamus/Pituitary	All of below
Thyroid	Pigmentation, headache, fatigue, etc
Adrenals	Acne, aging, fatigue, exhaustion
Pancreas	Acne, blood sugar imbalance
Ovaries	Acne, pigmentation, rosacea, aging, moodiness, PMS

Table 6: Imbalances in the endocrine glands and typical symptoms.

MELASMA AND STRESS

Stress is an everyday companion that can affect each of us in different ways. Exhaustion, feeling emotionally unwell, a rapid heart rate, tension, etc. are all responses from our body to stress factors in our environments. These responses are modulated by stress hormones that are produced and released by three of our endocrine glands – the hypothalamus, pituitary gland and adrenal glands. Though in our case, I should say four glands, since the skin has the ability to produce and release stress hormones as well. The fact that the skin has a stress response might not be so familiar to you, but we all experience stress responses from our skin, such as sweating, redness and swelling.

Below is a glossary of terms to understand the stress response. You do not have to study the terms first. Come back to the glossary once you have started reading the chapter.

CRH–corticotrophin-releasing hormone, released from the hypothalamus or skin cells after stress is perceived, induces a cascade of stress responses to endure the survival of cells

α-MSH–alpha-melanocyte stimulating hormone, released from the pituitary gland and skin cells, strong pigmenting effects, also connected to emotions

ACTH–adrenocorticotropic hormone, released by the pituitary gland and skin cells, derived from POMC after CRH is released, stimulates the release of cortisol in adrenals, strong pigmenting effects

Adrenaline–also called epinephrine, is the stress hormone that is released by the adrenal glands when a sudden stress factor occurs (attack or excitement), increased breathing and blood flow, also released by keratinocytes in the epidermis

Cortisol–is the stress hormone that is released by the adrenal glands when stress persists and adrenaline is weaned off, lowers inflammation

POMC–proopiomelanocortin protein, activated after the action of CRH; ACTH and α-MSH are derived from POMC

HPA axis–also called the hypothalamus pituitary axis or stress response

HOW THE SKIN IS LINKED TO THE STRESS RESPONSE AND THE ADRENAL GLANDS

The skin does not exactly belong to the endocrine system and is more recognised and known as an organ rather than a gland. But as mentioned in the previous paragraph, the skin can induce a stress response. Let me explain this. I will start with the systemic (body) stress response. One of the easiest-to-imagine scenarios of a stress response is the example of the attack from a sabre-toothed tiger when we were hairy and primitive sapiens. Imagine you, a few thousand years back as a primate walking around, foraging for food. All of a sudden you find yourself in a standoff with a sabre-toothed tiger, and you perceive that as a dangerous situation. Your body is noticing your emotion and instantly, within milliseconds, your endocrine glands will release stress hormones to help you run for your life. The body automatically reacts in this way to allow an increased blood flow to your muscles so you can run faster. This is only one simple example of a stress response and the purpose of stress hormones but there are several others. But what they all have in common is a sequence of steps that follow a certain pattern. Involved in this pattern are specific endocrine glands and stress hormones. The sequence of hormone release is as followed:

Stressor perceived » release of CRH from the hypothalamus » release of ACTH from the pituitary gland » release of adrenaline from the adrenals » if stress persists longer release of cortisol from adrenals after adrenaline reservoir is exhausted.

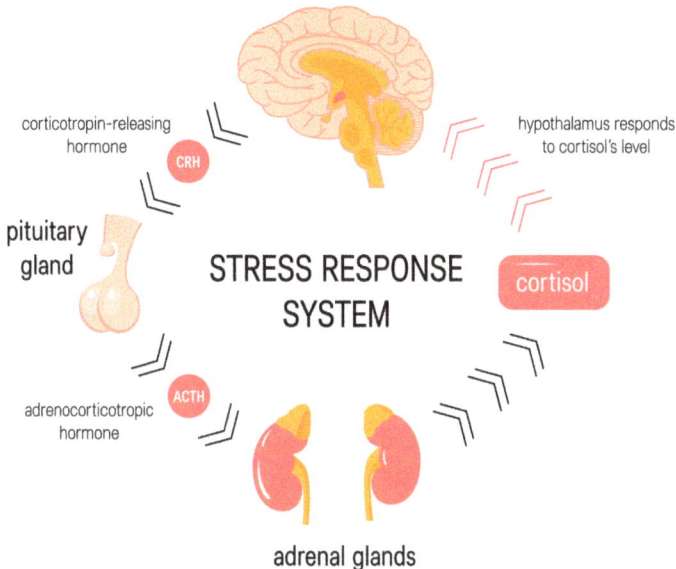

Image 10: Schematic view of the HPA axis (stress response) (Credit: marina_ua).

The body always follows this hierarchy from the hypothalamus to the pituitary gland and to the adrenals, which is called hypothalamus-pituitary-adrenal axis, or HPA axis for short. The main reason why the body is creating a stress response is to regain balance (homeostasis), which ensures survival, repair and protection. The stress hormone adrenaline, for example, increases blood flow to the muscles to move faster. Cortisol reduces inflammation to regulate the immune system. But stressors are not just of mental and emotional nature. Stressors can also be chemicals, physical pressure, radiation, microorganisms, etc., which are perceived by the HPA axis. And this axis also exists in the skin.

The skin acts as our barrier and gatekeeper to protect our inner world from the outside world and is often the first unit to come in contact with environmental stressors. One of the best-known skin stress responses is the sunburn caused by the stress factor ultraviolet radiation (as part of the sunlight) when enjoyed in excess amounts. To ensure a quick response to stressors, the skin has developed its own local stress response without having to wait for the body to activate its defence mechanisms.

Dr. Andrzej Slominski from the University of Alabama has dedicated more than three decades to the research of stress response and pigmentation. In the late 90s, he was the first to discover that the skin follows the same pattern in its stress response as the body (HPA axis) and has since published numerous papers on the topic [47][48]. The equivalent pattern followed by the skin is simply called the cutaneous (Latin for skin) or local HPA axis.

Furthermore, the stress response and the endocrine system of the skin are connected to the broader endocrine system. This means that if the body's system becomes activated, the skin can respond with symptoms and when the skin's endocrine system becomes activated, the body can respond with symptoms. The connection between the skin and the body's endocrine system has been felt by everyone who has experienced a decent sunburn. A sunburn is a stress response from the skin when too much sunlight is absorbed. You can probably remember that it can make you feel pretty crappy. Damage to the skin does not go unnoticed by the body. Feeling queasy after a sunburn forces you into rest mode, which is helpful to ensure optimum repair. The point I am making is that the skin is not a separate entity from the body and the body is not separate from the skin. But what has all that to do with melasma?

Skin cells in the epidermis and dermis can produce, release and respond to the same stress hormones the systemic endocrine glands produce and release to respond with repair and protection. The protection mechanism here is the tan that is created by the skin pigment melanin to protect the skin and body from future sunburns. Melanin is the brown pigment that appears after sun exposure and can absorb UV radiation to act as our natural sunscreen. Therefore, acquired skin pigmentation (tan) is a stress response. This is further explained when we discuss the function of stress hormones.

You have just learned that the tan is a stress response of the skin to ultraviolet light. But the stress response of the skin is not just activated by the sunlight. Any kind of stressor perceived by the skin can activate the skin's HPA axis. Pigmentation as a response within the HPA axis is mediated by stress hormones and these hormones are not picky about what stressor they respond to. Chemicals, loss of skin cells due to injury and even stored toxins and medications can have the same effects on that HPA axis as radiation from the sun. Ever had a dark mark after a scratch? That is pigmentation presenting as a stress response from a physical injury, meaning melanocytes have responded to the physical stress. Hyperpigmentation is a common result of injuries after laser treatments, peels or needling due to damage and inflammation. UV light is not needed to bring up a dark mark after a skin injury, but sun exposure would act as a catalyst and darken the mark to ensure protection. Pigmentation from injuries can fade but sometimes stay for a lifetime.

Since we know that the endocrine system of the body and the skin are connected, we can imagine that emotional and mental stress can affect our skin too. As melasma is often connected to the hormone estrogen, the connection to other hormones of the endocrine system is not surprising. Still, the medical and beauty industry does not always make the connection to stress when a patient or client concerned with melasma is seeking help for their current condition.

Our melanocytes possess receptors that respond to stress hormones. They cannot distinguish between hormones from neighbour skin cells or stress hormones from endocrine glands that have been released after experiencing emotional stress or ongoing overwhelm.

I know from experience when consulting clients that traumatic experiences often happened around the time of the onset of melasma. One of my clients reported to me her melasma appeared shortly after her dog passed away. Other clients have reported having very stressful jobs when their melasma came up. This may be anecdotal accounting, but there is supporting clinical evidence as well.

In 1987, the Department of Dermatology in Tel Aviv reported about two patients who developed Melasma 8–10 weeks after the death of two close relatives. The clinicians involved in the observation considered α-MSH, due to emotional stress, as the reason for the melasma outbreak [49].

In the following paragraphs, we will explore how the different stress hormones affect skin hyperpigmentation.

CRH

CRH is made in the hypothalamus and has the role of the starter hormone in the stress response and the pigmentation process by initiating the release of ACTH and α-MSH. CRH has another meaningful role in melasma as it builds a connection between the stress response and the immune system.

In 2005, a research team discovered for the first time that human mast cells respond to CRH. Mast cells are cells that are recruited from the immune system when the body is having an allergic reaction and they are linked to chronic inflammatory conditions. The team found that mast cells release vascular endothelial growth factor (VEGF) in response to CRH [50]. This means that the formation of new blood vessels, which typically occurs in melasma, could be a stress response with inflammation mediated by CRH and mast cells.

Professor Dr. Slominski, who focuses on the skin stress response and melanogenesis in his work states that mast cells have a special place in the brain and skin axis, as they play a significant role in the interaction between the immune and nervous system [51]. We will learn more about the link of melanocytes to VEGF and mast cells and why the formation of new blood vessels is a stress response in Part II, titled "Melasma and the Immune System".

α-MSH

The main function of the hormone α-MSH is the pigmentation of hair, skin and eyes, while it is also a member of the stress response. It belongs to the melanocortin system, which influences pigmentation, energy homeostasis and sexual function (the melanocortin system is also tightly connected to the thyroid, see "Melasma and the Thyroid"). α-MSH is typically elevated in pregnant women from the third trimester due to the release of CRH from the placenta and plays a major role in pregnancy-related melasma. This hormone is released by the pituitary gland, skin cells and nerve endings in the skin (typically after sun exposure) [52].

α-MSH originates from a protein called proopiomelanocortin (POMC). POMC is also the source of ACTH, which is the precursor of the stress hormone cortisol. POMC can be synthesised to α-MSH and ACTH. While the main function of ACTH is to stimulate the production of cortisol in the adrenals, it also exerts strong effects on pigmentation. Furthermore, if ACTH is not utilised to make cortisol, it can break down into α-MSH, like in Addison's disease with the consequences of skin hyperpigmentation as we will discuss shortly.

Skin pigmentation by α-MSH: Stressor » CRH production and release in hypothalamus or skin cells » POMC activation » α-MSH production and release in the pituitary gland or skin cells » α-MSH attaches to melanocyte » pigmentation

ACTH

Adrenocorticotropin (ACTH) is a hormone released by the pituitary gland that initiates a signal to your adrenals to produce cortisol, but it can also be produced by cells of the epidermis and dermis. How ACTH can impact skin pigmentation is demonstrated by several health conditions that impact the central HPA axis, such as Addison's or Cushing's Disease. People with Addison's disease have fatigued adrenals, which leads over time to less production of the stress hormone cortisol. This happens when people are in an ongoing state of stress and the adrenals cannot keep up with the demand of stress hormones. As a result, the feedback loop is disrupted, and the pituitary gland keeps releasing ACTH, as it does not receive cortisol as the signal to stop the release. The ongoing release of ACTH from the pituitary gland will over time lead to hyperpigmented skin.

There are two variations to how hyperpigmentation occurs. Number one is that increased ACTH from the pituitary gland breaks down into α-MSH (both are derived from POMC; increased POMC » increased ACTH/α-MSH). The other option is that the ACTH's ability to dock onto α-MSH receptors enables melanocytes to directly respond to ACTH with pigmentation. Freckles can show in earlier stages, while extensive hyperpigmentation appears in a progressed stage. Think of the skin colour of the ex-president of the United States Donald Trump. Do we really believe he is having weekly spray tans? The stress load of a president in the United States is humongous. Some people believe John F. Kennedy suffered from Addison's Disease as well.

And if we search for photos of both presidents and compare their skin tones from the start of their careers as politicians to the end of their legislature, we can see drastic changes in their skin pigmentation [53][54][55][56].

Addison's disease and melasma are of course not the same, but we cannot neglect the fact that hyperpigmentation is related to mental and emotional stress. And since we have not found solutions in the treatment for melasma, we have to look at the facts given and connect the dots that seem further apart. Let us look into the clinical research on how ACTH is affecting melanocytes. You will notice that the way ACTH impacts the behaviour of melanocytes is strikingly similar to how melanocytes behave in melasma.

A research team has documented how melanocytes become enlarged and more dendritic after incubation with ACTH from the pituitary gland. Under the same experimental conditions, ACTH also increased tyrosinase activity, which is also a feature of melasma [57]. Dendritic means melanocytes can reach more keratinocytes to "dye" the cells with melanin (dendrites look like tentacles as you can see in image 3). Both, the increased size and increased dendricity are hallmarks seen in melanocytes of melasma lesions. Tyrosinase is the enzyme that is needed to form melanin. That ACTH increases tyrosinase activity could be confirmed by two other studies from the late 90s. In both investigations, human melanocytes were incubated with ACTH. They found that ACTH had very potent effects on tyrosinase activity. These effects on the cells were observed without the use of UV light [58][59].

ADRENALINE

Adrenaline can directly induce melanin production. Adrenaline is the stress hormone that is released by the adrenals as the first stress response, when a sudden threat occurs (flight or fight response) and by keratinocytes in the skin. A research team in 2004 found that melanocytes are able to respond to adrenaline as they possess the adrenaline receptor ß2-AR. Melanocytes had more melanin after they were incubated with adrenaline [60]. This demonstrates that there is a communication between keratinocytes and melanocytes and an indicator that damage to keratinocytes can signal melanocytes to increase pigment production. Meaning that physical injury to the skin surface can cause pigmentation via adrenaline release (scratching, needle pricks, etc.).

It also means that circulating adrenaline has the potential to cause skin pigmentation. Adrenaline usually does not stay long in the system but is it possible that the constant release of this hormone after reoccurring stress triggers potentially induced hyperpigmentation? Also, adrenaline is used in medicine to treat anaphylactic shocks, cardiac arrest and asthma. It raises the question if the long-term use of these meds can potentially contribute to pigmentation. Furthermore, melanin can directly be derived from a hormone group called catecholamines, which includes noradrenaline, adrenaline and dopamine. These three hormones can be directly converted into melanin by the action of tyrosinase or metal ions. The ability of this conversion is based on their common origin from the amino acid l-tyrosine [2]. If we have increased levels of metal ions stored in our tissues and/or increased tyrosinase activity, is it possible that the stress hormone can be converted to melanin as consequence?

SUMMARY—MELASMA AND STRESS

Any form of stress perceived, if local on the skin or central to the whole body, can induce hyperpigmentation. Melanocytes are not able to distinguish between stress hormones perceived by skin cells and stress hormones released from the brain or adrenal glands.

• Stress hormones can stimulate pigmentation without UV light.

• Stressors that release stress hormones can be emotional stress, chemicals on the skin (acid, harsh cosmetics), radiation (sunlight, artificial light), toxicity from metals and medications or physical injury (a scratch, for example).

• CRH from the hypothalamus is the start hormone of every stress response, the precursor of α-MSH (alpha melanin-stimulating hormone) and stimulates mast cells to release VEGF [50]; VEGF increases blood vessel formation as seen in melasma patients.

• α-MSH is the primary hormone in the skin pigmentation process and closely related to the stress response.

• ACTH from the pituitary gland increases the size and dendricity of melanocytes [57] and increases tyrosinase activity [57][58][59]; those are typical features of melasma.

• Adrenaline increases the melanin content in melanocytes [60] and can be converted into melanin with tyrosinase and metal ions [2].

A REMARK ON MELASMA AND STRESS

Even though we know that the sun is a stressor and can be the cause of hyperpigmentation, we must consider all stressors to be a factor in the development of melasma. Melasma has become a much bigger problem in the past ten years. I have made this observation when diagnosing skin of thousands of people for the past 15 years. The sun has been with us since the beginning of time but our modern lifestyles have birthed stressors that have been with us for less than a century. Don't get me wrong, humans had tough times in many aspects 100 years ago, but now we face a life where we perceive constant mental and emotional stress and we are more exposed to environmental toxins.

Modern technology, like cell phones and computers, are new advances, and likely, our physiologies have not caught up to adapt to their impacts. Hence, we are constantly overtaxing our systems. We receive phone calls, emails and other requests all at the same time and are always urgent while remaining sitting still at our desks. Sound familiar? There is no running away from these threats as back in the old days when we encountered sabre-toothed tigers. The stress can go nowhere else other than the body where it disrupts the delicate balance, resulting in exhausted adrenal glands.

Additionally, the expectations of performance have increased with new technologies. Having a hands-free work meeting while driving the kids to school is considered to be no problem. Multi-tasking is worn as a badge of honour. We have included synthetic chemicals in our daily lives. We ingest them, we apply them to our skin, we wear toxic clothes, we sleep on toxic mattresses and cook our food in toxic pots and pans. We hide from natural sunlight and expose ourselves to artificial light all day well beyond daylight hours. Our bodies were not designed to cope with most modern stressors we are exposed to, with the result being an overly activated central and local stress response.

We discuss all the possible stress factors in Part III and provide solutions in Part IV.

MELASMA AND THE THYROID

Changes in the skin, especially in pigmentation, are not uncommon and are well reported in patients with thyroid dysfunctions. Overactivity of the thyroid, also called hyperthyroidism, is often associated with hyperpigmentation, as seen in Graves' disease (an autoimmune condition) [61][62]. On the other hand, underactivity of the thyroid, also called hypothyroidism, is often associated with hypopigmentation (lack of pigment) like the skin condition vitiligo. This skin condition is not uncommon to appear in patients with the thyroid autoimmune condition Hashimoto's disease. The irregular pigmentation in vitiligo typically appears in a symmetrical pattern and extensive patches, similar to melasma. I will explain how pigmentation and the thyroid are related.

Below is a glossary of terms to give you a glimpse into the different thyroid hormones. You do not have to study the terms first. Instead, come back to the glossary once you have started reading the chapter to solidify the information and terms used.

TRH–Thyrotropin releasing hormone produced in the hypothalamus

TSH–Thyroid stimulating hormone produced in the pituitary gland, stimulates T3 and T4 production in the thyroid

TPO–Thyroid peroxidase, an enzyme that uses iodine to make it usable for T4 and T3 production, is stimulated by TSH

T4–Free thyroxine, released by the thyroid, a prohormone of T3

T3–released by the thyroid, regulates thyroid function

abTG–Anti thyroglobulin–an antibody against thyroglobulin-thyroglobulin is a peptide that is needed for T3 and T4 synthesis, 3–40 nanogram per ml is normal. High levels can be a sign of the autoimmune conditions of Grave's disease or Hashimoto's disease.

Anti-TPO–antibodies that stop TPO from using iodine (can be a sign of Hashimoto's disease)

HOW THE SKIN IS CONNECTED TO THE THYROID

The interaction between the hypothalamus, pituitary gland and thyroid is called the hypothalamus-pituitary-thyroid axis (HPT axis). The HPT axis interacts with the melanocortin system, which is the main regulator of human skin pigmentation [63].

The melanocortin system consists of melanocortin receptors (e.g., melanocortin receptor-1), which sit on melanocytes, and the corresponding hormones ACTH and α-MSH. The system is involved in metabolism, skin pigmentation, stress response and fight or flight response. The interaction of the melanocortin receptor-1 (MC1R) and the hormones ACTH and α-MSH is significant in regard to pigmentation and the thyroid connection. ACTH and α-MSH are both hormones involved in melanogenesis (synthesis of melanin) and produced by the pituitary gland and skin cells (e.g., after sun exposure). Sometimes, the pigmentation process goes awry and is a symptom in response to an imbalance in our health, rather than a natural process. Now here is where it becomes a little bit more complicated.

The melanocortin system itself is orchestrated by two groups of neurons in the hypothalamus. Those neurons can synthesise two different proteins that are crucial in the pigmentation process but also have a direct influence on the thyroid. Those two proteins are POMC and agouti-related protein. POMC activates the TRH production in the hypothalamus as the starter for thyroid hormone production. And POMC is also the precursor of α-MSH and ACTH, the hormones that activate pigmentation. The other protein mentioned, the agouti-related protein, has the opposite effect to POMC and can inhibit pigmentation and TRH activity [64][65]. Agouti-related protein is often mentioned in correlation with the hypo-pigmentary condition vitiligo. Vitiligo is linked to an underactive thyroid, as well as thyroid-related autoimmune states, and as mentioned before also has a symmetrical pattern with more extensive patches like melasma. Do you see the link? The connection of the neuron-derived proteins POMC and agouti-related protein to the HPT axis and the melanocortin system is additional evidence of how tightly the skin is connected to the inner systems of the body.

A great example of how pigmentation and the thyroid are connected can be envisioned when we look at the effects of the so-called "Barbie drug" Melanotan. People have it injected under their skin to get skinnier, more tanned and to increase their libido. The active ingredient of Melanotan is a synthetic version of the melanocortin hormone alpha melanocyte stimulating hormone (α-MSH). The effect is a faster metabolism and deep tanning of the skin. Melanotan is not regulated and is illegal in most western countries but is apparently still sold in beauty parlours and fitness centres and is available to buy online. The use of this promising wonder drug can come with unpleasant side effects, such as the appearance of moles and freckles, nausea, vomiting, loss of appetite, flushing of the face, involuntary stretching and yawning and spontaneous erections [66]. Some of the symptoms resemble the symptoms of hyperthyroidism, such as increased metabolism and increased body temperature.

Research suggests that the melanocortin system is more likely to impact the HPT axis, rather than the HPT axis affecting the melanocortin system. A trial on rats demonstrated that α-MSH has a role in activating the TSH gene and increasing the circulating levels of free thyroxine (T4) levels [67]. Another trial on rats showed that injection of α-MSH into their brains increased plasma TSH [68]. This means that hyperpigmentation in melasma is not necessarily the result of a dysfunction in the thyroid but that pigmentary changes in the skin can be a sign and warning that there is an overactivity in the nervous system. We can assume that a disturbing factor is arousing the production of proteins and hormones in the brain that as a result affects skin pigmentation and thyroid function.

The following studies I am going to present, demonstrate the commonality of changes in thyroid hormone levels in melasma patients.

A study from 1985 with 108 women, demonstrated a 4-fold higher incidence of thyroid dysfunction in melasma patients compared to their control group with no melasma. Also, 70% of the women who reported a link between the onset of melasma with pregnancy or contraceptives, had a thyroid dysfunction. Melasma patients with idiopathic causes (cause not known) had a 40% rate of thyroid dysfunction. The incidence of thyroid dysfunction in subjects without melasma was only 12.5% [69].

Another study from 2015 enrolled 70 women with melasma and compared them to a control group of women without melasma (none of them pregnant). The researchers found that 18.5% of melasma patients had thyroid disorders, while only 4.3% of subjects from the control group had thyroid issues. Furthermore, 15.7% had positive anti-TPO (thyroid peroxide antibodies, a sign of Hashimoto's disease), whereas only 5.7% in the control group (without melasma) had positive anti-TPO [70].

In a study conducted in Iran with 45 melasma patients and 45 control subjects, 24.4% of melasma patients had higher anti-TPO than average. Only 6.7% of people in the control group had elevated anti-TPO levels [71].

A Turkish study from 2015 included a group of 45 women with melasma and a control group of 45 women without melasma. T4 (free thyroxine), TSH (thyroid stimulating hormone) and AbTG (anti-thyroglobulin) levels were all significantly higher in the melasma group compared to the control group (Table 7) [15].

PARAMETER	PATIENT GROUP (MEDIAN ± SD)	CONTROL GROUP (MEDIAN ± SD)
T3 (pg/ml)	2.98 ± 0.45	2.94 ± 0.37
T4 (ng/dl)	1.16 ± 0.19	0.99 ± 0.19
TSH (mlU/ml)	2.36 ± 1.24	1.72 ± 0.99
abTG (IU/ml)	44.9 ± 9.69	32.04 ± 8.23
abTPO (IU/ml)	20.8 ± 5.7	30.08 ± 10.67
Presence of thyroid nodules, n (%)	12 (26.7)	15 (33.3)
thyroid parenchyma, n (%)	4 (8.9)	2 (4.4)

Table 7: Example of thyroid levels in melasma patients [15].

SUMMARY—MELASMA AND THE THYROID

- There is a 4x higher incidence of thyroid dysfunction in melasma.

- TSH, T4, abTG and anti-TPO are elevated in melasma patients.

- The system involved in pigmentation (melanocortin system) is tightly linked to the Thyroid axis (HPT axis).

The results of the research on melasma and thyroid dysfunction indicate an autoimmune response and elevated thyroid hormone levels. But what do we do with these results? What drives thyroid antibodies in melasma patients? According to many holistic clinicians, diet, environmental toxins and emotional trauma are the main contributing factors to thyroid dysfunction. Dr. Wentz, a pharmacist and a Hashimoto patient herself, states that she sees a significant correlation between autoimmune-related thyroid conditions and two major factors. One is diet, where patients can improve their health within days of implementing specific dietary changes. The other factor is experiencing times of great stress, which she could recall as a factor in the onset of her own Hashimoto journey [72].

Thyroid hormones originate from the hypothalamus and pituitary gland in the brain. When thyroid hormone levels in melasma patients deviate from normal levels, then shouldn't we consider the regulation and balancing of the hypothalamus and pituitary gland as a practical approach to treating melasma patients with thyroid dysfunction? If so, then it is worth enquiring what is responsible for imbalances in the brain.

In the previous chapter about stress and melasma, I mentioned a study from Israel where researchers assumed that α-MSH due to emotionally traumatic events was causative to the development of melasma [49]. We know excess ACTH can break down into α-MSH, resulting in hyperpigmentation. Both pituitary hormones, ACTH and α-MSH, are inseparable from the thyroid. This means that a response of the thyroid to stress with the consequence of hyperpigmentation (or hypopigementation) is very probable. Furthermore, a chronic excess of thyroid hormones (T3 and T4) in the system causes inflammation [73] [74]. Inflammation is a common coexisting factor in melasma, which we will find out soon.

MELASMA AND ESTROGEN

The sex hormone estrogen is speculated to be the main causative factor in melasma, as it often shows up in pregnant women or women who use the contraceptive pill. It is therefore also called the "mask of pregnancy". The effects of estrogen on hyperpigmentation have been well studied but are not yet completely understood. In the following text, we explore the connection between hyperpigmentation and estrogen. Later in Part III, I will present a myriad of reasons that increase estrogen levels.

HOW ESTROGEN IS LINKED TO HYPERPIGMENTATION

Melanocytes respond to the sex hormone estrogen via their corresponding receptors. When an estrogen molecule docks onto an estrogen receptor (sitting on the cell surface of the melanocyte), the melanocyte becomes animated to induce melanin production. More specifically, melanocytes become larger and more dendritic when in contact with estrogen (estradiol – E2, estriol – E3 and progesterone) [57].

Estrogen also increases the activity of the melanin-converting enzyme tyrosinase [75]. The effect of estrogen on the pigmentation process can typically be seen in the darkening of the areolas and vertical line that forms below the belly button during pregnancy. Also, the contraceptive pill is known for its estrogenic effects on skin pigmentation.

But, melasma is an emerging problem among women who have neither been pregnant nor have undergone any hormonal treatment, including birth control pills. In my daily work over the past 17 years, I have observed that the pill and pregnancy cannot be the only cause. This observation is confirmed if we look at the data presented in Part I, "Demographics", on how melasma patients assess their onset. Although many surveys confirm that pregnancy and contraceptive pills play a role in the development of melasma, the numbers also reveal that these factors are not covering the entire spectrum of this pigmentation disorder.

A study in Pakistan evaluated the hormone levels of 150 women with melasma; none were pregnant or using oral contraceptives. Still, 89% had elevated estrogen, and 55% had deviations in progesterone levels [18].

A survey in Brazil investigated trigger factors of melasma in 300 women. In response to the survey, 36% of women confirmed pregnancy as an onset factor, while 16% of women reported the contraceptive pill as their trigger [12].

An international investigation about trigger factors was conducted on 324 melasma patients, where patients from 9 different skin clinics reported their triggers via questionnaire. While 42% of women said their onset date was during pregnancy, only 25% of melasma patients claimed that melasma appeared for the first time after the use of oral contraceptives [14].

	PREGNANCY	CONTRACEPTIVE PILL
300 WOMEN [12]	36%	16%
324 WOMEN [14]	42%	25%

Table 8: Women who suspect the onset of melasma due to pregnancy or the contraceptive pill.

The data raises questions about the correlation between melasma and pregnancy or the contraceptive pill when only 42% of melasma patients connect their onset to pregnancy, and a maximum of 25% of women reported taking the contraceptive pill as an onset event. Even though this is a significant percentage, there is no doubt that other factors must be considered contributory to elevated estrogen levels. And it raises the question of what these factors are.

Also, should melasma not subside once the pregnancy hormones drop or the contraceptive pill is stopped?

Many of my clients who reported their onset time of melasma to be correlated to their pregnancies or using the pill cannot get rid of their melasma even many years after.

Another evidence that pregnancy and the pill are not the only causes of elevated estrogen is the fact that men can be affected by it. Several papers confirm the occurrence of melasma among our male population. The percentage of men with melasma in an Indian study was 20% [1]. So, what is the reason for elevated estrogen that causes melasma to appear in women and men if pregnancy and contraceptive pills can be ruled out?

Factors that raise estrogen levels:

1. **Blocked pathways of estrogen elimination** (e.g., poor liver function)
   The liver digests all fat-soluble substances in the body, including fat-soluble hormones, such as estrogen. Suppose the liver has to work too hard to metabolise other substances, such as fat from the diet or alcohol and medication. In that case, estrogen will stay stored in the liver, which leads to an accumulation of estrogen. Read about factors in Part III, "Medication", "Heavy Metals", and "Diet, Food Additives and Pesticides", and in Part IV ", Detox from Heavy Metals", "Food as Healer", and "Supplements as First Aid" for holistic solutions.

2. **High stress**

   Read more about factors in Part III, "Emotional Stress and Trauma", and find solutions in Part IV, "Reducing Emotional and Mental Stress".

3. **High blood sugar** (high sugar diet, including alcohol)
   Find more about the effects of sugar on estrogen in Part IV, "Refraining from Certain Foods and Food Additives".

4. **Excess weight**
   Fat tissue is known to be a primary site of estrogen production and additionally favours the activity of estrogen synthesising enzymes (aromatase) [76][77].

5. **Copper toxicity**
   Find more details in Part III, "Heavy Metals – Copper", and solutions in Part IV, "Detox – Heavy Metals".

6. **Gut microbiome dysbiosis**
   The gut is taking part in the estrogen metabolism. After the liver breaks down estrogen, the estrogen metabolites are carried to the gut, where they are either eliminated with the stool or reabsorbed and recirculated through the body. Particular gut bacteria that are called the estrobolome, excrete a specific enzyme (beta-glucuronidase) that converts estrogen into its active form for reabsorption. When there is an imbalance in the gut microbiome, and estrobolome takes over, too much active estrogen is reabsorbed, which leads to increased estrogen [78].
   Find more details in Part III, "Imbalances in the Gut Microbiome".

7. Low fibre diet
   Fibre in your diet is needed to eliminate hormones.

8. Disrupted circadian rhythm
   Find more details in Part III, "Artificial Light".

9. Endocrine disruptors
   Find details in Part III, "Endocrine Disruptors".

10. Mold
    Read more in Part III, "Mold".

11. Oral contraceptives and other estrogen-containing medications

FOOLED HORMONE RECEPTORS

Apart from excess estrogen, another possible factor that could cause the body to react atypically to estrogen is the receptor response. A cell can respond to a hormone with higher intensity when the sensitivity and number of the hormone receptors are increased. The more receptors are available, the more sensitive the cell will be to the hormone. Increased receptor sensitivity to estrogen in melasma-affected skin was found to be true in a small trial for the first time in 2008. The small trial was conducted on biopsies of two subjects and could prove the increased expression (increased quantity) of estrogen receptors on melasma skin compared to non-lesional skin [79].

Other studies confirmed an increase in hormone receptors in melasma skin to be a contributing factor. The investigation was conducted on 33 women, and the parameters were more specific. The research team was not only testing the estrogen receptors but also progesterone receptors. They tested for cell receptors in the epidermis and dermis. The result was that the epidermal lesions showed no increase in estrogen receptor expression but in progesterone receptor expression. The melasma lesions in the dermal layer showed an increase in estrogen receptor count but not in progesterone receptor levels [80][81].

Some hormone replacement medications, which are widely used to prevent or treat breast cancer, can confuse the hormone response of cells. Tamoxifen, for example, reduces estrogen levels by blocking and inactivating the estrogen receptors in breast tissue (antagonistic action). However, the drug can act differently in other tissues, for example, occupying the receptor and increasing the response of the estrogen receptor (agonistic action). If you read through the forums on the internet, you will find that melasma is a quite common side effect among tamoxifen users. I also had a client who was on tamoxifen and showed melasma-like hyperpigmentation on her upper cheeks. An in vitro trial could confirm that tamoxifen can induce pigmentation in epidermal melanocytes. The research team was interested in the repigmentation of grey hair with tamoxifen. They proved an increase in melanin after melanocytes were incubated with the drug [82].

It seems contradictory that women who use this drug complain about dark spots. Given that hyperpigemtation is likely to occur with elevated estrogen levels, while tamoxifen should have an anti-estrogenic effect. But we do not yet know how this drug acts on epidermal tissue. For example, tamoxifen acts on breast tissue as an antagonist, which means it lowers the response of the cells to estrogen. But on the other hand in genital tissue, it acts as an agonist where the drug promotes the response of cells to estrogen and therefore benefits the development of cancer [83].

Tamoxifen was found to increase estrogen production in the ovaries of premenopausal women [84]. It is suspected that the long-term use of this drug can have estrogenic effects as opposed to the anti-estrogenic effect [85]. Two case reports present clinical records of women who experienced melasma after using tamoxifen (both after breast cancer surgery). One patient reported having noticed the brown patches after she had used tamoxifen for a month [86].

Another woman studied had vitiligo and reported a complete depigmentation of her face after chemotherapy for breast cancer treatment. She was given tamoxifen, and five days after using it, brown patches on her cheeks started to appear [87].

SUMMARY—MELASMA AND ESTROGEN

- Estrogen enlarges melanocytes, increases their dendricity and increases tyrosinase activity.

- Pregnancy and the contraceptive pill are not the only causes of elevated estrogen. Other factors like endocrine disruptors, stress and other environmental and lifestyle conditions play a part (See Part III).

- Disrupted estrogen receptors affect the estrogen response with potential impacts on skin pigmentation.

Our modern lifestyles contribute largely to elevated estrogen levels. Numerous environmental toxins and medications, chemicals in cosmetics, metals in our foods and drinking water, not to mention stress, can confuse our hormone system. These choices promote behaviours and diets that are not ideal for our health, and stress levels are skyrocketing. Endocrine disruptors play a big part in the confusion of our hormone system as they can mimic hormones and block receptors. As we found out, those disruptors can include medications, but there are many potential disruptors like metals, BPA and mold, which are discussed in Part III, "Environmental Toxins".

SUMMARY—MELASMA AND THE ENDOCRINE SYSTEM

All hormones released by endocrine glands rely on signals from the brain, the hypothalamus and the pituitary gland. Could it be that hormonal imbalances are dysfunctions in the pituitary gland, as it is the master gland that all hormones originate from? Is balancing and healing the pituitary gland the solution aspect we need to focus on?

Our clinical research has come so far, yet we are still at the beginning of exploring the magnitude and complexity of the human body's physiology. Thus far, research cannot provide a clear conclusion on the connection between melasma and the endocrine system. Regardless, we do know that hormones have significant effects. It is not necessary to know the exact and detailed molecular connections to get the idea that hormone health and balance are critical for well-being and healthy skin. What we can take from the chapter about the endocrine system is that we should become conscious of our daily habits, possible threats and stressors, whilst making daily changes and improvements to help us become healthier.

MELASMA AND THE IMMUNE SYSTEM

A SHORT INTRODUCTION

In this chapter, we will explore how the immune system and inflammation are related to skin pigmentation. I will also present evidence of inflammation in instances of melasma. But first, a bit more on the immune system and pigmentation.

The immune system is your body's defence mechanism to fight threats such as microorganisms, stress and toxins. Conversely, it also initiates the healing processes of the damage caused by those threats. It is also engaged when the body's nervous and endocrine systems are out of balance. Several organs, bones, blood, lymph and skin are all part of the immune defence. Once the body has sensed a threat and the immune system is alerted, immune cells are recruited to the place of emergency via the bloodstream where they release peptides and heal the damage.

The skin is the first line of defence against threats and an indicator of an activated immune system. Indicators of an activated immune system are often visible on the skin as rashes, itchiness, redness and swelling. The redness and swelling are caused by peptides and are immune markers like cytokines and histamines, released by immune cells. When immune markers are present, the body is in an inflammatory state.

The skin can respond to the systemic immune system but has its own local immune system to react immediately to threats like chemicals on the skin. When threats like environmental toxins overwhelm our bodies, our systems become out of balance and the immune system is trying to regain this balance. Deficiencies can also cause the immune system to be in a state of imbalance. For example, when we lack a mineral or vitamin, we are more open to reacting to environmental threats such as microorganisms and are more prone to infections.

We can have a deficiency of:

- a nutrient (vitamin or mineral)

- an antioxidant

- air (oxygen, carbon dioxide or carbon monoxide)

- gut bacteria

Or toxicity of:

- a chemical (food, water, air, etc., e.g., heavy metals, pesticides)

- free radicals

- a pathogen (bacteria, virus, fungi, parasite)

- a hormone (sex hormones, stress, etc.)

- or too much stress; emotional or physical

» Imbalances alert your immune system and cause inflammation in your body.

MELASMA IS AN INFLAMMATORY SKIN CONDITION

There is considerable evidence of a link between melasma and the immune system. An Iranian study revealed a correlation between the inflammatory skin condition "post-inflammatory hyperpigmentation (PIH)" and melasma. The study involved 400 study subjects. They compared 200 women with melasma and acne with 200 women who had acne but no melasma. A dermatologist evaluated the presence of post-inflammatory pigmentation in both groups. The melasma patients were nearly three times more likely to develop post-inflammatory hyperpigmentation from acne (66.8%) compared to the group with acne but no melasma (24.1%) [88]. This data from patients who suffer from melasma and acne gives precious insight into the inflammatory potential of melasma. But how does inflammation cause pigmentation?

When skin pigmentation appears darker than your usual skin tone after the impact of a stressor like sun exposure, you have an immune response from your skin to protect itself. In other words, hyperpigmentation is an immune response (as well as a stress response as we discussed in the chapter "Melasma and Stress"). Sunburn, for example, is inflammation resulting from an immune response due to excess sun exposure. The inflammatory response is mediated by the action of immune cells and inflammatory markers, such as cytokines. Immune cells release specific cytokines that activate melanocytes after trauma on the skin.

Skin traumas that evoke pigmentation can be burns, scratches or even breakouts, as in the case of post-inflammatory hyperpigmentation. Hyperpigmentation after a scratch, for example, is the result of an acute stressor with acute inflammation. The intention of the body is to protect the trauma site from more damage, which could potentially occur if the wound would be exposed to UV light. The melanin within the trauma area acts as natural protection. The pigmentation usually fades once the inflammation has subsided along with the healing of the wound. Melasma is hyperpigmentation that is persistent as it is the result of chronic inflammation from a chronic stress factor and I will explain the details as followed.

The skin responds to acute or chronic inflammation as well as acute or chronic stress. Acute stress causes the immune system to respond with acute inflammation (e.g., scratch or sunburn). Chronic stress can cause the immune system to respond with chronic inflammation (e.g., psoriasis or melasma). Chronic inflammation occurs when your body is repeatedly exposed to relatively small stressors, such as the daily baring of our lives to air pollution and pesticides, as well as toxins in textiles and cosmetics. This continuous susceptiveness produces a steady, low-level inflammation throughout the body, which damages overall health and can lead to longstanding pigmentation that is hard to get rid of.

As mentioned earlier, when the immune system is triggered, specific immune cells are recruited, and inflammatory markers are released by cells to fight the stressor. As long as the stressor persists, the immune system will continue to release cytokines. Those stressors are environmental toxins, which we are constantly exposed to. As a result, we live in a chronic state of low-grade inflammation with the potential result of skin problems, such as melasma. I will present the evidence, which is documented in numerous studies as followed.

HOW IMMUNE MARKERS CAN CAUSE HYPERPIGMENTATION AND MELASMA

Immune markers can be different cells and cell fragments in the blood and other tissues when threats are present. The immune cells and markers that were found in melasma lesions include mast cells, lymphocytes and cytokines. Cytokines are protein fragments of the immune system that serve as signalling factors and their presence is a clear indicator of inflammation.

SCF

A cytokine identified as stem cell factor (SCF) was repeatedly found in the skin samples of melasma patients. SCF is secreted by fibroblasts and keratinocytes; it plays a critical role in normal skin pigmentation. SCF functions as a survival mechanism for melanocytes; for example, after a skin injury, such as sunburn. SCF is released when fibroblasts from the dermal layer or keratinocytes from the epidermal layer have been damaged. SFC then sends a signal to the melanocytes in the epidermal layer to activate the protection mechanism pigmentation [89] [90][91].

A Korean study from 2006 examined skin samples of 60 women with melasma. They compared skin samples of melasma and non-melasma lesions in the epidermis (location of melanocytes and keratinocytes) and dermis (location of fibroblasts). They found a significantly higher level of SCF expression in the melasma lesions compared to melasma-free samples in the dermal layer. There was no difference in the SCF expression in the samples of the epidermal layer [92].

This means that the SCF was released by fibroblasts and not from keratinocytes, which confirms the significance and involvement of the dermis and fibroblasts in the development of melasma. This gives more insight into the healing approach for the skin and shows us how our skin layers are connected to each other.

Particular pathways support the connection and communication between skin layers and cells [90][93][91]. I imagine them like phone cords enabling fibroblasts and melanocytes to talk to each other. The connection between the different skin layers has the benefit of repair and renewal, but it also means that when one layer of the skin is wounded, another layer of the skin is affected too.

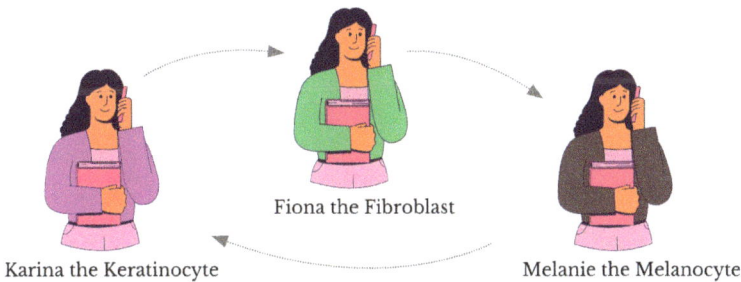

Fiona the Fibroblast

Karina the Keratinocyte

Melanie the Melanocyte

Image 11: A metaphorical depiction of skin cell communication.

It is normal to find SCF in the dermis after extended sun exposure as a normal immune response to stress. After radiation, the skin is geared to induce melanin production to give you a tan and protect you from radiation. But UV is not the only factor that can stimulate fibroblasts in the dermis to release SCF. Any kind of stress can trigger the release of inflammatory markers. Several studies confirmed the release of SFC after UV exposure, but this does not automatically mean that other factors are not causing cytokine release. Laboratories usually use UV light to mimic an inflammatory response in the skin because it is an easy-to-apply and approved method. This often leads to the assumption that the factor that was chosen as a methodical parameter to prove a reaction is the only factor to consider. Also, note that in clinical research environments, the skin is often exposed to excessive amounts until blistering. Yet, this is not a common situation in people's daily lives. Also, UV lamps are not imitating the sunlight in its true and natural state. While UVB and UVA rays are often separated in research settings, UV lamps can also emit damaging UVC rays.

In medicine, SCF is used to treat people with certain blood conditions. The pigmenting effect of SCF is demonstrated in case studies conducted without UV light exposure after cytokine injections in the skin. In some cases, SCF injections have caused hyperpigmentation on the injection site and presented cosmetic problems for patients [94][95]. An activating effect of SCF in melanocytes was also confirmed by an in vitro experiment, where melanocytes were injected with SCF. No UV light was used. The melanocytes became activated and enlarged after injection [96]. Another study from 2018 reported that SCF alone, without UV, can stimulate melanogenesis in human melanocytes [97]. We explore possible factors that trigger SCF release in Part III.

LYMPHOCYTES

In 2005 a research team investigated changes in the skin of 21 melasma patients. They took skin samples and found an increased lymphocyte count in 75% of melasma-affected samples. The melanocytes were enlarged and very dendritic, which increases the transfer of melanin to surrounding skin cells [6]. Lymphocytes are white blood cells (also known as B and T cells) whose presence in tissues is a clear indicator of inflammation. They are typically recruited to fight off infections and toxins.

MAST CELLS

A research team in Mexico evaluated skin samples of 27 patients with melasma. They found that mast cells were much more prominent in melasma lesions than in healthy skin [98]. An increased mast cell count is an indicator of allergic reactions and inflammation. Mast cells are located in organs directly connected to the outer environment, like lungs, skin and gut. They are recruited after contact with triggers like air pollution, pollen, food additives, medication or venom. Could the increased mast cell count in melasma indicate a reaction to a toxin, allergen, air pollution or pesticides?

Mast cells secrete several cytokines, such as SCF and VEGF (VEGF is needed to produce new blood vessels). You might remember from Part I that one of the typical features of melasma is an increase in VEGF and blood vessels around the markings. We will find more evidence on VEGF in melasma and the factors responsible for it in Part III, "Air Pollution".

LEUKOTRIENES AND THROMBOXANES

Mast cells also synthesise the cytokines leukotrienes and thromboxanes. Those are the type of inflammatory markers that are expressed when chronic inflammatory conditions are present. They are recruited when the skin, lungs and gut perceive threats such as allergens and are present in the lungs of asthma patients or the skin of patients with atopic dermatitis. These cytokines are also known to stimulate the pigmentation process. In 1992 an in-vitro study found that melanocytes become more dendritic and swollen, and tyrosinase increases when cultured with leukotrienes and thromboxanes [99][100]; those features coincide with the features of melanocytes in melasma.

Leukotrienes are derived from cell membrane lipids; they form after cell membranes have broken down (lipid peroxidation). Lipid peroxidation typically happens when cells experience oxidative stress. Oxidative stress is an imbalance of antioxidants and free radicals where free radicals have the upper hand. Melasma represents precisely the same features that appear when leukotrienes are present: increased size and dendricity of melanocytes, increased tyrosinase activity, impaired barrier function and disrupted basement membrane (likely as a result of cell membrane breakdown).

COX-2

More evidence of inflammation in melasma comes from a Mexican study. An increase of COX-2, an enzyme that indicates inflammation, was present in skin samples of 20 melasma patients (they also found increased levels of lymphocytes, mast cells, macrophages and the cytokine interleukin-17) [101]. COX-2 is needed to form leukotriene from cell membrane lipids. Its action is induced in response to oxidative stress [102].

It is likely that toxins in our environment cause oxidative stress in our skin cells, which subsequently causes the release of COX-2. We will soon find out more about oxidative stress, the link to melasma in "Melasma and Oxidative Stress" and contributing factors in Part III.

HISTAMINES

Histamines are another product of immune cells that act on melanocytes. They are important chemicals in the allergic response and are secreted by mast cells. They are released by mast cells when the immune system has detected an allergen from food or air, for example, and trigger typical allergy reactions, such as increased blood flow to excrete the toxin. Histamines were subject to a clinical trial to examine their pigmentation potential due to the presence of mast cells in melasma and other skin disorders of pigmentation, such as urticaria pigmentosa. The outbreak of the latter skin condition is usually triggered by food, heat and certain medications. In vitro studies have demonstrated that histamines increase tyrosinase activity, increase the size of melanocytes and make them more dendritic [103][104].

SUMMARY—MELASMA AND THE IMMUNE SYSTEM

- Immune cells, such as mast cells and lymphocytes, and inflammatory markers, such as SCF, interleukin-17 and COX-2, are present in melasma lesions.

- Patients with acne and melasma are three times more likely to develop post-inflammatory pigmentation than acne patients without melasma.

- VEGF, released by mast cells, is present in melasma and forms new blood vessels; a typical feature of melasma.

- Leukotrienes, released by mast cells, can induce lipid peroxidation and increase tyrosinase activity, which are features of melasma.

- COX-2 is an indicator of lipid peroxidation.

- Histamines released by mast cells can induce pigmentation and change melanocytes into a melasma-typical morphology.

It is undeniable that hyperpigmentation and melasma are tightly linked to inflammation. There is evidence of inflammation based on the presence of mast cells, lymphocytes, SCF, leukotrienes and histamines in melasma and hyperpigmented skin. Those immune cells and markers point to a reaction caused by environmental stressors, such as allergens, toxins in our food and air and maybe even infections. We explore the possible stress factors in detail in Part III and offer holistic solutions in Part IV.

MELASMA AND OXIDATIVE STRESS

AN INTRODUCTION

Oxidative stress is another imbalance in the body that is linked to melasma. The body is in a state of oxidative stress when there is an imbalance in the antioxidant and free radical exchange of cells. Oxidative stress can induce cell morphologies that are typical in melasma-affected skin. It can break down healthy cell material, such as cell membranes (lipid peroxidation), cause inflammation, and evoke pigmentation as a protection mechanism.

HOW OXIDATIVE STRESS OCCURS

Imbalances in the free radical and antioxidant ratio can happen due to internal processes, such as cell metabolism and external factors, such as air pollution or environmental toxins. Some examples of cell metabolism processes are the exchange of nutrients and waste products in and out of the cell, cell breathing, the production of new cell material, as well as the healing process when inflammation is present.

In the example of cell breathing (or cell respiration), the goal is to produce energy for the cell and to maintain homeostasis. This happens in the mitochondria (singular = mitochondrion) of each of your cells small cell organelles that are working hard like an engine every single second. Without a mitochondrion, there can be no life. The tasks a mitochondrion has to do require enzymes as catalysts produced within this cell organelle. Some of those enzymes act as antioxidants and are therefore able to neutralise free radicals (not all antioxidants have enzymatic activity).

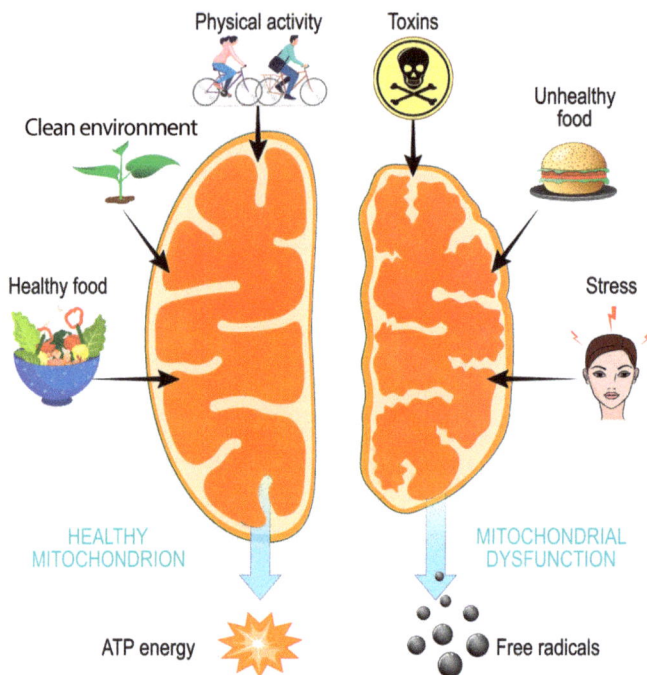

Image 12: How oxidative stress impacts the mitochondria (Credit: ttsz & Collette Sadler).

Free radicals are also called reactive oxygen species (ROS) or nitrogen oxygen species (NOS), depending on their chemical composition. Cell breathing creates waste products similar to how the body digests and excretes waste from the food we eat. The cells do the same thing, just on a micro level.

Free radicals can be categorised as endogenous and exogenous. Endogenous free radicals are waste products formed during cell metabolism. Exogenous free radicals are formed in our outer environment because of the earth's breathing and recycling system. Even though free radicals have a negative connotation as a threat and scavenger, they are also needed, and their purpose is to destroy pathogens along with breaking down cell material in our bodies.

Free radicals are built with an unpaired electron in their atomic structure, which is an unstable state. As atoms are geared to achieve an atomic neutral balance, free radicals tend to attach to other atoms, which can compromise their stability (Image 13). This often leads to a cascade of damage if atoms of molecules have no spare electrons to donate. Antioxidants are coming in as saviours as they possess donor electrons, enabling free radicals to attach to them and abrogate their harmful potential. Consequently, free radicals only become harmful if we lack antioxidants to neutralise them. When this is the case, we experience oxidative stress.

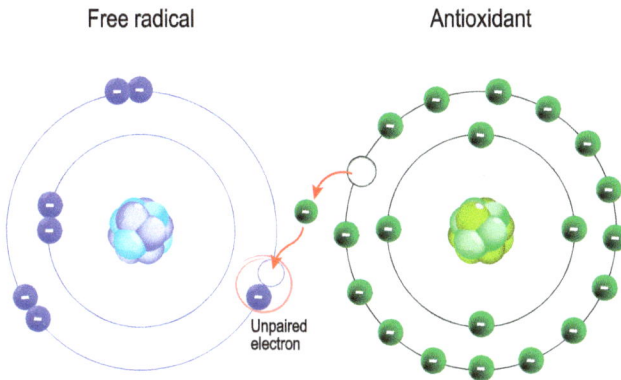

Image 13: The electron exchange between free radicals and antioxidants (Credit: ttsz).

We can receive antioxidants from plants (exogenous antioxidants) in addition to our own antioxidants (endogenous). Most of us might be more familiar with antioxidants from foods, such as vitamin C from fruit. Still, our body's antioxidants hold an immense power of protection and healing potential.

Some of the primary antioxidants produced in your mitochondria are:

- CoQ10

- NADH

- Glutathione

- Alpha-lipoic acid

- Bilirubin

- Ferritin

- Superoxide dismutase (SOD)

- Catalase

- Glutathione peroxidase [105]

WHY OXIDATIVE STRESS IS HARMFUL

Oxidative stress describes the state of an imbalance between free radicals and antioxidants in the body. If there are not enough antioxidants available, free radicals will attack healthy cells to gain a neutral state. This causes disturbance in the homeostasis of our cells and can subsequently lead to cell damage or premature cell death. Toxins from the diet, cosmetic products, radiation and environmental pollution are foreign to the natural environment in our cells. They can cause an overload of waste products and, therefore, disturbances in the free radical and antioxidant balance with the consequence of the depletion of cell material, such as the lipids of the membrane (lipid peroxidation). As a result, the cells die, the skin becomes thinner, and the barrier is impaired. As we remember from Part I, a thinned epidermis and a disrupted basement membrane are typical features of melasma.

A healthy lifestyle should maintain homeostasis in our cells with no oxidative stress, but modern living conditions cause an imbalance and accelerate natural cell death, even in our younger years.

THE EVIDENCE OF OXIDATIVE STRESS IN MELASMA

Research has found that oxidative stress is involved in the development of melasma. The findings revealed that an accumulation of free radicals goes along with an increase in melanin. The reason is that melanin is a natural antioxidant and therefore scavenger of free radicals and appears to protect melanocytes from the toxic effects of ROS [106]. This means that if free radicals are dominant, melanocytes respond with increased pigmentation to neutralise the damaging effects. Also, oxidative stress is a common cause of inflammation, which we have learned is linked to melasma.

The Cutaneous and Ocular Toxicology Journal published an article in 2013 that measured antioxidant and free radical levels in melasma patients. The study involved 50 patients with melasma and 50 subjects as a control group. They found that the balance between free radicals and antioxidants in the skin with melasma was significantly disrupted compared to the control group [107].

A research team in India measured the levels of endogenous antioxidants and oxidative stress in patients with melasma compared to a control group. They found that the serum levels of the endogenous antioxidants melatonin and catalase were significantly lower among the melasma cases compared to controls. The serum levels of protein carbonyl (a marker for oxidative stress) and the endogenous free radical nitric oxide were significantly higher in cases compared to controls [108].

Another research team detected an increased amount of the enzyme nitric oxide synthase (iNOS), which is part of nitric oxide formation, in skin samples of melasma patients [109].

Nitric oxide is a molecule in our atmosphere and bodies. It can act as a free radical and antioxidant. Nitric oxide (NO) benefits the body; it supplies oxygen to the cells and plays a part in the natural skin pigmentation process. The production of NO usually happens after UV radiation in keratinocytes and promotes pigmentation. Nitric oxide's effects on pigmentation are increased tyrosinase activity [110] and more dendritic melanocytes [111]. Increased tyrosinase activity and increased dendricity of melanocytes are both features of melasma lesions.

SUMMARY—MELASMA AND OXIDATIVE STRESS

- An increase of free radicals (oxidative stress) is present in melasma.

- Increased melanin is the result of high levels of free radicals as melanin acts as a neutraliser (antioxidant).

- High levels of free radicals induce typical features of melasma, like increased lipid peroxidation, tyrosinase activity and melanocytes with more dendricity.

The production and presence of free radicals in our inner and outer environment are normal and even needed. Still, if we do not have the antioxidant resources to neutralise those, we risk damaging precious cell material in a state of inflammation. Our modern lifestyles have brought forth many factors, including increased exposure to air and food toxins, which can lead to excessive amounts of free radicals that our bodies cannot handle. Additionally, unhealthy lifestyle choices inhibit cellular function and compromise the health of mitochondria that produce most of our scavenger-neutralising antioxidants. As mentioned before, melanin acts as an endogenous antioxidant with neutralising effects of ROS to protect melanocytes from the toxic effects [106]. This elucidates a positive aspect of the overproduction of melanin when cells are in a state of oxidative stress, as it is a protective mechanism in favour of the cell. Unfortunately, this built-in protection comes with unwanted cosmetic outcomes.

As nitric oxide assists the oxygen supply, it begs the question if the presence of increased nitric oxide can also be a sign of oxygen deprivation in melasma. Could it be that environmental stressors deprive the skin of oxygen, and the increase of nitric oxide is an attempt of our body to flood the malnourished parts of the skin with oxygen to avoid cell death? Oxygen deprivation could also explain why increased blood vessel formation is a typical feature of melasma lesions since blood vessels are the vehicle of oxygen in the blood. And the increased oxygen supply to ensure cell survival could result in increased pigmentation as a side effect since oxygen plays a vital part in the pigmentation process.

The factors that cause oxidative stress are outlined in Part III. Ways to reduce oxidative stress, increase mitochondrial health and how to activate endogenous antioxidants will be discussed further in Part IV.

MELASMA AND GENETICS

Our genes play a critical part in our physiological functions. Without them, no biological process could happen. We inherit our genetic make-up from our parents, which determines our looks, but can also predispose us to specific health conditions. In Part I, we discussed that up to 65% of melasma patients had reported a positive family history. Often, we hear that having specific genes predispose us to disease; therefore, we are left with the belief that we must accept the fate of our genes. But whether we develop the same health conditions as our parents depends on our environment. Thanks to the work of Bruce Lipton from Stanford University, who birthed the field of epigenetics, we now know that genes are active or inactive, depending on the environment our cells live in.

In other words, we can manage our genetic predisposition if we don't trigger specific gene expression (activity) by environmental factors like foods, thoughts and other lifestyle choices. You are not doomed to develop melasma because of your genetic make-up. The human genome (the sum of all your genes) has not changed in thousands of years. But what has changed is the environment and lifestyle of many. This needs to change again for the better if we want to become healthy. The environment you surround yourself with, the macrocosmos, and the environment your cells are embedded in, the microcosmos, are of great significance for your health. This means if you create an ideal outer and inner environment for your body, genes predisposed to cause disease might never get activated and, therefore, will not lead you down a path of illness.

WHAT CHINESE FACE READING CAN TELL YOU ABOUT MELASMA

Chinese Face reading is 5000 years old and is used as a diagnostic tool in Traditional Chinese Medicine (TCM). In ancient China, doctors were not allowed to see female patients undressed. To examine and diagnose patients, doctors had to rely on changes and specific signs in the face and pulse to diagnose disease. The idea of seeing internal disease on the outside is not far-fetched. When we buy fruit and vegetables, we assess the outside marks and blemishes to determine if the fruit is tainted inside. We humans are not so different from fruit and vegetables in that regard. In TCM, each part of the skin is associated with a specific organ or gland, as seen in the image below.

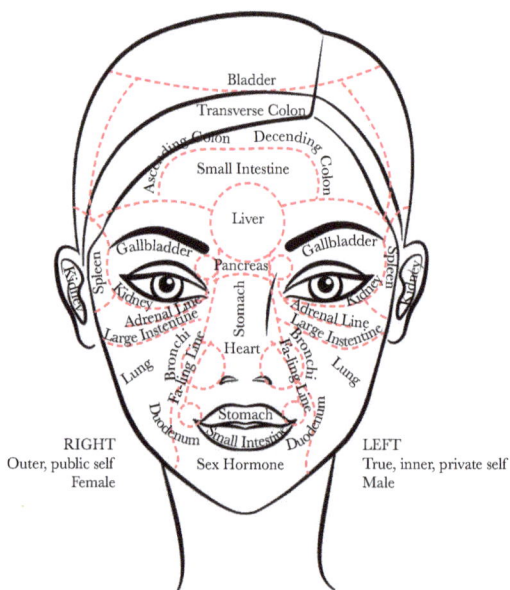

Image 14: A face map that portrays where organs and glands are showing up in the face according to Traditional Chinese Medicine. (Credit: juliawhite & Collette Sadler)

The parts of the face that interest us the most are the ones where melasma appears, specifically the forehead, the nose, the upper and lower cheeks, the upper lip and the chin. You can see how the location of melasma marks on the face is linked to the system's organs. Some possible factors that disturb the organs are also included. We will explore more of the factors in Part III.

LOCATION OF MELASMA LESION	CORRESPONDING ORGAN	POTENTIAL HEALTH ISSUE
Forehead	Colon and Small Intestine	Gut microbiome dysbiosis Irritating foods and food additives
Nose	Heart and Stomach	Irritating foods and food additives Emotional stress
Upper cheeks	Large Intestine	Irritants in the digestive system Gut microbiome dysbiosis
Lower cheeks	Lungs	Air pollution
Upper lip & chin	Sex organs	Sex hormone imbalance (e.g., estrogen)

Table 9: Interpretation of potential internal issues in relation to the location of melasma lesions.

Book recommendation:

"WTF? Why the Face" by Dr. Todd Frisch

A REMARK TO PART II

We dove into the physiology of the body and learned how vastly interwoven the web is between the skin and our body's internal environment. We know that melasma does not only appear in pregnant women and women on contraceptive pills but also does not disappear easily. We have learned how stress, thyroid imbalances, inflammation and free radicals play a role. When the nervous or endocrine systems are out of balance or we experience oxidative stress, we trigger the immune system. These disruptions can trigger an uneven pigmentation response, often reinforced by the sun. The takeaway of Part II is that an imbalance of the systems is causative and correlated to melasma and that homeostasis is crucial for health and wellbeing.

The insights we have gained from Part II also offer a different perspective on the healing approach. When we look at the correlation between inflammation and melasma, we can conclude that every treatment option that induces more inflammation should be avoided. That means no laser or other treatments that reach into the dermis and cause damage and inflammation (temporarily or permanent) to the skin should be a treatment choice for melasma.

PART III

THE FACTORS THAT CAUSE IMBALANCES

In the previous Part II, we explored the clinical evidence on how melasma is correlated to imbalances in the nervous, endocrine and immune systems as well as oxidative stress. In Part III, we will open our minds to various environmental factors that explain why imbalances in our bodies occur. Those environmental factors are the reason why melasma has become more prevalent in modern times.

EMOTIONAL STRESS AND TRAUMA

Can cause:

- an activated nervous system with an increase in nerve growth factor (NGF)

- disruption of the endocrine system

  - increase of ACTH due to desensitisation of cortisol [112]

  - correlation of childhood trauma and pituitary dysfunction [113][112]

  - increase of stress hormones » estrogen dominance

- autoimmune-related conditions, e.g., Hashimoto's disease [114]

- inflammation

- oxidative stress

- production of endogenous free radicals [115]

The word stress is a broad term for a myriad of everyday pressures. We first sense emotional stress in our hearts and minds but eventually feel it in our bodies and see it on our skin. Emotional stress arises for many different reasons; for example, when we think that we have not met the expectations of ourselves and others, when the workload and responsibilities become too much, when we experience losses and separations or when we feel we have lost control.

If you have melasma, you certainly know that this itself causes distress as it affects the face and is therefore easily visible and constantly present in everyday life. Do you feel it negatively impacts your life's quality and psychological and emotional well-being? Have you searched for a dermatologist or other skin therapists only to find they could not resolve the problem? Have you experienced feelings of shame, low self-esteem, lack of joy and felt unmotivated to go out?

You are not alone. The tragic reality is that even suicidal ideas are not uncommon among melasma patients [5].

We might not like to acknowledge this, but emotional stress affects women more intensely than men (check out the work of Dr. Legato on gender medicine) [116]. I say this because women have worked hard to attain equality in the past 100 years. However, being vulnerable and sensitive is not a weakness and does not damage the hard-earned achievements of emancipated women. We can choose to embrace our femininity and tenderness with pride. It is the trait that men admire us for, and that makes women sensitive carers for children and the vulnerable. We do not have to pretend to be emotionally resilient like men to be respected as an equal in society. We must learn to set boundaries and say no in our most feminine and vulnerable voice. We can be strong and still acknowledge that we are sensitive. We do not need to adapt to masculinity to be able to respond to men and to measure up to the expectations that were brought forth by the patriarchal world.

If we constantly try to bend and adapt beyond our natural and feminine flows, we overtax our nervous systems, disrupt the endocrine system and negatively affect our immune system. Chronic and persistent stress confuses the stress response over time, resulting in adrenal fatigue. Cortisol levels become depleted, cortisol secretion is reduced, and the receptors become resistant or decrease in number. It is known that people with post-traumatic stress disorder (PTSD) show decreased levels of cortisol [117]. Over time, depleted cortisol levels lead to an overproduction of ACTH in the pituitary gland, which can result in skin pigmentation (adrenal fatigue » ACTH increases » skin pigmentation). Remember in Part II, "Melasma and Stress", the cases of women who experienced melasma after significant losses.

The negative effects of chronic mental and emotional stress on our systems will sooner or later show up on our skin. If it has already come in the form of melasma, please do not ignore the signs and instead expand your choice of treatment beyond the application of cosmetics. Everything you have learned in the chapter about melasma as a stress response can be applied to emotional stress as a factor. Enquire within yourself to understand your own personal story and whether the melasma outbreak correlates to emotional stress. You will find some guidance for self-enquiry in the questionnaire in the appendix. The connection between melasma, the thyroid and the immune system is also linked to emotions.

Emotional stress is now becoming accepted in medicine as a cause of autoimmune conditions, such as Hashimoto's disease. A large cohort study with over 15,000 patients with autoimmune disorders was conducted to assess a correlation between autoimmune conditions with childhood trauma. The traumas included as parameters were physical, sexual and emotional abuse, as well as witnessing domestic violence, substance abuse, mental illness and divorce. It was found that 64% of all participants experienced at least one of those qualifying events [114].

One of the purposes of the stress hormone cortisol is the suppression of the immune system and reduction of inflammation. When we experience ongoing stress, our cortisol reserves become depleted. It is therefore not surprising that we find our immune system activated and our body chronically inflamed in a state of perpetual stress.

Also, childhood trauma is believed to cause pituitary gland dysfunctions later in life, which can affect the whole endocrine system and sexual hormone secretion. This observation was made when researchers found that severe childhood trauma is a common event in patients with pituitary tumours [112]. It was also found that children who experience violence or sexual abuse reached puberty at an earlier age [118][119]. Earlier onset of puberty means the earlier onset of sex hormone production, which begins in the pituitary gland. By no means do I venture to say that everyone who suffers from melasma or thyroid dysfunctions or both had endured such traumas. But I want to raise awareness of how far dysfunctions in the endocrine system reach and encourage you to develop a deeper understanding of human physiology. The deeper we dig, the deeper our healing journey can unfold.

Let's circle back to the question of what raises estrogen levels. There is a connection between stress and estrogen dominance. When the body is depleted of cortisol reserves to cope with stress, the source of new cortisol is the sex hormone progesterone. This decreases progesterone levels. When progesterone is decreased, estrogen becomes dominant. Whether estrogen dominance is affecting melasma is not confirmed, since estrogen dominance and elevated estrogen levels are not particularly the same thing. But since we know that stress hormones can cause hyperpigmentation directly and because imbalances of one hormone affect the entire endocrine system, stress reduction should always be part of a healing protocol.

You will find solutions for pituitary health and emotional trauma in Part IV – "Heal and Nourish – Reduce and Heal Emotional Stress".

ENVIRONMENTAL TOXINS

Can cause:

- a confused endocrine system

- oxidative stress [115]

- an overactive immune system

- inflammation

- disruption in the gut microbiome

Endocrine disruptors, medication, food additives, pesticides and mycotoxins from mold are typical environmental toxins in our daily lives. Some are manufactured, like synthetic pesticides, while some occur naturally, such as mold (fungi). You might wonder why those substances are a problem for our health and if they really are dangerous. We must understand that every substance ingested, absorbed and inhaled by the body goes through a digestive cycle to utilise nutrients and neutralise toxins. This process causes cells to produce waste products (e.g., free radicals) and metabolites, which are eventually excreted. The more chemicals we are exposed to, the more of these waste products we produce. As we have learned in Part II, "Melasma and Oxidative Stress", if we cannot neutralise free radicals with antioxidants, we are in a state of oxidative stress.

Let us look at the number of environmental toxins we are exposed to on a daily basis. It does not surprise that our bodies are in a constant state of imbalance, oxidative stress and chronic low-grade inflammation. Some of those toxins, like endocrine disruptors, are very powerful in mimicking hormones and disrupt the endocrine system. Others, such as pesticides cause inflammation and oxidative stress. Let's dive into the topic and explore the research.

ENDOCRINE DISRUPTORS

Can cause:

- a confused endocrine system

- oxidative stress » increased lipid peroxidation [120][121]

- inflammation [121][122]

Most endocrine disruptors (ED) are manufactured chemical compounds found in our environment and homes. They are in our cosmetic products, carpets, tap water, cleaning products, food, food containers, etc. They are not easy to completely avoid, but we can reduce them and minimise the risk of exposure if we know what to look out for. Even small amounts of endocrine disruptors can have big effects on our delicate hormone system. The World Health Organisation (WHO) knows about the negative health effects of ED. Their official definition is: "… an exogenous substance or mixture that alters function(s) of the endocrine system and consequently causes adverse health effects in an intact organism, or its progeny, or (sub)populations." [123].

The NIEHS, an association dedicated to the research of ED and health hazards, has identified ten different key characteristics of ED [124]. Endocrine Disruptors can increase or lower hormone release by attaching to hormone receptors and either inactivating the response (antagonist) or increasing the responsivity (agonist). When an endocrine disruptor acts as an agonist, it mimics a hormone and acts as a fake hormone activating the response of the cell. Let us take the example of ED as an agonist and the potential effect on estrogen receptive cells (like ovarian, breast or skin cells) to explain the outcome of such a response.

When the ED acts as fake estrogen and attaches to the estrogen receptor, it seems like the receptors are saturated, and estrogen production can stop. Unfortunately, because the particle attached to the estrogen receptor is fake, the glands receive the wrong message. As a result, the ovaries produce more estrogen because the real estrogen cannot attach to its receptor as someone else is already plugged into them. The pituitary gland in the brain does not receive the right message from the ovaries that there is enough estrogen already. Hence, it keeps sending the message to the ovaries to produce more hormones.

If this sounds confusing and chaotic to you, it's because it is! Furthermore, ED can alter hormone receptor expression, which changes the sensitivity of the cell to respond to hormones. We have evidence that estrogen receptor expression in melasma is altered (see Part II – "Estrogen"). Another problem with ED is that they accumulate in the body and are not as easily excreted as actual hormones; therefore, they can impact how hormones are processed and eliminated. They can cause DNA damage and change the fate of the cell that produces the hormone or responds to the hormone (fate = cell death, development and division). Furthermore, ED cause oxidative stress and inflammation.

BPA, PBDE (flame retardants), phthalates and atrazine are some of the endocrine disruptors present in our environment. They are correlated with increased inflammatory markers interleukin-17 and COX-2 [122]. Those are the same inflammatory markers found in melasma (Part III – "Immune System"). The array of abilities an endocrine disruptor can perform is quite astonishing. Only a few of them are presented in this book, but as you know, they should be avoided if possible. There are plenty of alternative products to choose from, and products containing ED add no value to our lives and can cause harm.

The Environmental Working Group (EWG) released a list of "The Dirty Dozen" of endocrine disruptors.

"THE DIRTY DOZEN"

BPA – was considered for use as a synthetic estrogen in the 1930s [124], now found in all hard plastics and register receipts (ink)

Dioxin (PCBs) – herbicide production, waste burning, paper bleaching, found in animal products

Atrazine – a herbicide found in drinking water and crops

Phthalates – in most plastic, fragrances, building materials, kids' toys

Perchlorate – a byproduct of the aerospace, pharma and weapon industry – found in water

Fire retardants – in carpets, mattresses, dust, furniture, electronics, building materials

Lead – a heavy metal found in red lipstick, cacao, soil, drinking water

Arsenic – found in drinking water

Mercury – a heavy metal found in seafood (more under "Metals" in this part)

Perfluorinated chemicals (PFCs) – in non-stick cookware

Organophosphate Pesticides – neurotoxin developed in WW2 as chemical weapon, technologylater used as a pesticide

Glycol Esters – cleaning products, cosmetics, paint [125][126]

Additional ED to be aware of for nail polish lovers:

Triphenyl Phosphate (TPHP) – found in nail polishes from OPI, Sally Hansen, Wet 'n' Wild [127]

While some ED are banned these days, not all of them are because certain industries have not found, created or cared to create a replacement for them yet. And despite the ban on certain ones, they still remain in our environment because they are either part of building materials or simply cannot be broken down biologically – ever. Facts about the history and use of ED can absolutely evoke anger, as it illuminates the insanity of our modern world. This should not devastate us, but rather motivate us to take our health into our own hands and become activists.

Check out the below websites for more information on endocrine disruptors:

- ntn.org.au - many valuable links

- TEDX.org

- EDC-Free Europe

- Environmental Working Group, also available as an app

- http://www.ecospecifier.com.au huge database for safe consumer products

- Find solutions in Part IV.

MOLD

Can cause:

- endocrine system disruption due to mimicking of hormones

- an overactive immune system » inflammation

- disruption in the gut microbiome

Mold belongs to the fungi kingdom (no plant and no animal), thrives in moisture (like mushrooms in damp parts of the forest), and grows on food and surfaces. While mushrooms also belong to the kingdom of fungi and are very beneficial for our health, molds are seen as pathogens (disease-causing organisms). We know them from spoiled foods or water damage in the house (green, pink and black mold).

Molds can be absorbed through the skin, ingested or breathed in. They can interfere with our health directly or due to their secreted toxins. The toxins secreted by mold, also called mycotoxins, can damage the nervous system and DNA, shut down mitochondria, alert the immune system (excretion of cytokines and histamines from mast cells), cause oxidative stress and act as fake estrogens (myco-estrogens).

Mycotoxins activate the immune system and induce an inflammatory response by activating mast cells, which release cytokines and histamines [128][129]. The symptoms are similar to allergies with runny noses, itchy and red eyes, sneezing and coughing. Additionally, when we have mold toxicity, an oversensitivity to household items such as cleaning products, perfumes, smoke, glues, paints and cosmetic products is very common [130]. Other symptoms of mold toxicity can include brain fog, fatigue, anxiety and even depression [130][131].

Black mold from the species *Stachybotrys chartarum* produces the mycotoxin zearalenone, which is particularly known to interfere with the endocrine system due to its estrogenic impact. The toxin is mainly found in grains like corn, coffee and chocolate. The effect of zearalenone on the endocrine system garnered attention in the USA during the 1920s when a swine farmer noticed infertility in his female pigs after they were fed moldy grains [132]. Zearalenone resembles estradiol (E2), can bind to estrogen receptors and can exert estrogenic effects. Synthetic equivalents of zearalenone are still given to livestock to fatten them up and are used in pharmaceuticals to help women with postmenopausal symptoms [133].

Mold spores are natural competitors of bacteria. *Penicillium* is a genus of mold that has been widely used as an antibiotic (penicillin) since its discovery by Dr. Fleming in the late 1920s. We take advantage of Penicillium's ability to fight bacteria that make us sick. Still, since we are aware of the need for bacteria in our gut to maintain a healthy immune system, we know that this organism can disrupt our gut health. This is also true when we ingest molds from spoiled foods (blue-green, white, yellow and pink mold). In the chapter "Medication", we will learn that hyperpigmentation is linked to antibiotics (antibiotics are *Penicillium* derived). The effects mold and its toxins have as endocrine disruptors and on inflammation is an additional reason to consider this as a possible triggering or contributing factor for melasma.

Where do we find molds and mycotoxins?

- grains, especially maize (corn), barley, wheat, oats, rice and sorghum (can be contaminated with zearalenone, heat stable up to 160° Celsius) [134]

- low-quality coffee and chocolate

- spoiled foods

- water-damaged buildings and furniture

MEDICATIONS

Can cause:

- a confused endocrine system

- toxicity and inflammation

- a disrupted gut microbiome

Tetracycline and Minocycline are antibiotics used for acne and rosacea, which reportedly cause hyperpigmentation after long-term use. Iron chelates in the drugs are suspected to be responsible for the pigmentary reaction. The muddy brown pigmentation can become permanent or fade and resembles the look of poorly applied makeup [135][136].

Evidence shows a high binding affinity of various drugs to melanin. It is believed that melanin serves as a tissue protector from harmful toxins and chemicals and therefore holds onto drugs and chemicals stored in cells. The ability of drugs to retain pigment is not unknown since drug testing of hair samples is based on the principle of melanin as a binding agent. Melanin, in its physical structure, is an anion, which means it has negative polarity. This feature explains the affinity of melanin to bind to cations, such as metals and certain drugs (like chlorpromazine, which is an amine-cation) [137].

In the 1960s several reports emerged about drugs and chemicals that cause skin hyperpigmentation as a side effect. These drugs are still used today, and numerous recent case reports confirm a correlation to hyperpigmentation. Some of the alleged pharmaceuticals are used as treatments for depression, schizophrenia, bipolar disorder, OCD, malaria, rheumatoid arthritis and even nausea as well as chronic hiccups (chlorpromazine, chloroquine, and clomipramine are the names for the active agents) [137][138].

In 1964 a mental institution in Canada published a case study of eight patients where those treated with chlorpromazine showed skin hyperpigmentation. The clinicians reduced the hyperpigmentation in their patients by using two treatment approaches. One method was the chelation of copper to inactivate the tyrosinase activity, and the other was to increase melatonin in the body. Another interesting aspect of this report is that they mention the sudden death of five patients with hyperpigementation, whose autopsy revealed severe pigmentation in the kidneys, liver and lungs (please review "What Chinese Face Reading Can Tell You About Melasma") [139].

It is believed that chlorpromazine changes the metabolism of the amino acid tyrosine in the adrenal glands. Tyrosine is the amino acid that is used for melanin and adrenaline production. When the adrenals do not utilise tyrosine for adrenaline synthesis, the excess tyrosine is converted to melanin with UV as a catalyst [140]. It is reported that patients who use chlorpromazine have lower adrenaline levels, which indicates an excess of tyrosine. It was also reported that the pigmentation of patients who used chlorpromazine was found in the dermal layer. It is believed that melanin tends to drop into the dermis when melanocytes become exhausted. Also, the drug is attracted to melanin and stays trapped in the dermal layer, which makes drug-induced hyperpigmentation longer-lasting [140]. Furthermore, drugs that interfere with adrenal hormones can disrupt the feedback loop in the endocrine system. If a drug has an anti-stress hormone action in the adrenals, this can likely increase the α-MSH production in the pituitary gland, which stimulates skin pigmentation.

We shall not forget the birth control pill and other medications that contain estrogen as a possible factor due to the estrogenic action, which we have discussed in Part II.

Tranexamic acid is a medication regarded as a promising relief from melasma. It is an antifibrinolytic drug usually used in cases of heavy bleeding to inhibit plasmin formation. The hope with this drug is that it could reduce the blood vessel count, which is feeding the melasma lesions with oxygen and therefore creating more pigment. It is also suspected that tranexamic acid can inhibit melanogenesis due to the plasmin-blocking property, as plasmin has stimulatory effects in the formation of α-MSH [141]. The administration of this medication showed a reduction in the melanin content of melasma lesions, but it was observed that melanin increased in the skin around the lesions [142]. This is another example of how we create more imbalance if we do not address the root cause. Tranexamic acid showed improvement in symptomatic areas, but it worsened the healthy tissue. Thus, we must address the reason for the increased vessel count, instead of just reducing the vessel count.

DIET, FOOD ADDITIVES AND PESTICIDES

Can cause:

- an overactive immune system

- inflammation

- a disrupted endocrine system

- autoimmune conditions

- a leaky gut and gut inflammation

- excess estrogen from a high sugar diet

Food is not directly linked to hyperpigmentation, but our foods can be some of the most inflammatory factors in our daily life. Dr. Mark Hyman is an advocate of Functional Medicine and is a true believer that food is medicine. He supports the idea that corn, wheat and soy are the 3 top most inflammatory foods and should be avoided to reduce systemic inflammation. Many nutritionists and health practitioners believe that food sensitivities happen not because of the food itself but sensitivity to chemical additives and pesticides. Soy, corn and wheat used to be high-priority staple foods of the Asian, European and Native American people for thousands of years without problems of food allergies, leaky gut and chronic inflammation. Eating these foods is as old as the hills, but what has changed drastically are the farming practices and food preparation methods.

We must consider that our food can be laden with pesticides, antibiotics, heavy metals and other endocrine disruptors. Synthetic pesticides are endocrine disruptors and damage our gut flora. One particular pesticide, called paraquat, is correlated to hyperpigmentation. In 1980 Taiwanese paraquat manufacturers reported hyperpigmentation (and skin cancer), especially on sun-exposed areas of the skin [143]. Even small amounts can be highly toxic, and paraquat is banned in 32 countries (including most of the EU) but still heavily used in the USA, India, Australia, New Zealand and other countries [144][145][146]. Unfortunately, pesticides find their way into livestock, freshwater and aquatic animals. Once it is sprayed onto pastures, it is hard to control the intake of those chemicals by grazing cows and goats.

If the right foods are chosen, they can be a healer for your entire body. Find solutions and suggestions to improve gut health in Part IV, along with a list of the most common food additives to avoid in the appendix.

IMBALANCES IN THE GUT MICROBIOME

Can cause:

- disruption in the nervous system

- disruption in the endocrine system and high estrogen

- an overactive immune system

- inflammation

The subject of the gut microbiome (gut bacteria) is of great importance for melasma as it affects the nervous, endocrine and immune systems. To visualise the role of bacteria in humans, consider that the number of microbial cells in and on our body outweighs the total number of our body cells by ten times (we have trillions of cells in our body). The idea of bacteria on and in our body is frightening to some of us, considering we have been conditioned to believe that bacteria make us sick and that sanitising ourselves and our environment saves our children and us. The truth is, without bacteria, we would not survive. The gut directly communicates with the endocrine, nervous and immune systems.

Furthermore, the gut, brain and skin are organs that are active participants in the communication and regulation between these systems. Therefore, we cannot separate skin health from gut health and its microbiome. The connection of the gut, brain and skin (also called the gut-brain-skin axis) stems from the common origin of these organs during our time as embryos, which we discussed at the beginning of Part II. Our microbiome modulates the communication between the brain, gut and skin. Even small changes in the microbiome can cause inflammation in the body. One of the factors that cause changes in the gut microbiome is emotional stress.

In 1930, dermatologists John H. Stokes and Donald M. Pillsbury hypothesised that emotional states (e.g., depression and anxiety) could change intestinal microbiota, increase intestinal permeability, and contribute to systemic inflammation [147]. More than 100 years later, we know that emotional states can impact gut bacteria because hormones can change the microbiome and vice versa; bacteria can produce and secrete hormones [42]. With the gut microbiome, we now have one more piece of the puzzle to complete our mosaic of the interconnection between our skin and the rest of our body. The research that links hyperpigmentation directly to gut health is still minimal. However, the link between skin conditions like acne, psoriasis and atopic dermatitis and irregularities of the gut microbiome is well proven and documented.

Clinical research delivered evidence by examining the stool of patients and the success of treating skin conditions with oral probiotics. The success is attributed to the regained balance in the immune system, reduced inflammation and improved skin barrier. Factors other than emotions and hormones that change our microbiome are antibiotics, pesticides, medications, ingested toxins, alcohol and wrong or non-diverse diets. Healing the gut microbiome should be considered a primary approach in treating this inflammatory and hormone-related skin condition. You will find suggestions for solutions in Part IV.

HEAT, CHEMICALS AND PHYSICAL STRESSORS

As discussed in Part II, any stress on the body and skin evokes the release of stress hormones and inflammatory metabolites, which can subsequently provoke skin pigmentation. Cosmetic treatments such as peels, laser and needling are the latest trends to fight skin aging, scarring and pigmentation. These treatments involve the removal of skin cells deeper than an ordinary facial scrub. The results of such impact on the skin can deliver astonishing results but pose risks such as hyperpigmentation from potential injury. Therefore, they belong in the hands of qualified practitioners with a high level of education and responsible behaviour.

HEAT

A Chinese study has found that laser treatments can cause hyperpigmentation. The stimulation of fibroblasts after treatments with laser (The Q-switched frequency-doubled Nd: YAG 532nm laser) caused the secretion of cytokines (e.g., SFC, HGF and bFGF), which the research group suspected as the reason for increased melanin after the treatment. Unfortunately, an increase in collagen, which was the aim of this laser treatment, could not be detected [148]. We have discussed the pigmenting effects of SCF in Part II, "Melasma and the Immune System".

CHEMICALS IN COSMETICS

Chemical peels with Trichloroacetic acid (TCA) have a strong ablating effect on the skin and can lead to unwanted hyperpigmentation. A study has confirmed that this effect is caused by the skin's stress response in an effort to regain its homeostasis and heal the wound. They found that keratinocytes express POMC protein after the peel [149]. We have learned in Part II, "Melasma and Stress", that POMC is the trailblazer for the stress hormones ACTH and α-MSH, which can directly induce skin pigmentation.

PHYSICAL STRESSORS

There are risks involved with all treatments that cause physical injury to the skin. Treatments like microneedling where your epidermis and even dermis are pricked with very fine needles can improve the skin for some people who suffer from scarring, pigmentation or those who want to achieve more firmness. A lot of other people who have had such treatment reported regret from damaged skin. People with genetically dark skin (from Fitzpatrick III and over) are especially prone to develop hyperpigmentation after more invasive treatments that cause short-term inflammation. You have to decide for yourself if you want to take the risk; there is no guarantee of success. But I beg you to stay away from special deals from questionable places.

AIR POLLUTION

Can cause:

- oxidative stress

- insufficiency of oxygen in tissues (hypoxia) » SCF release » increased blood vessel formation

- overactivity of the immune system » inflammation

Air pollution is linked to hyperpigmentation and melasma due to a chemical reaction in the skin after the absorption of nanosized airborne particles (air pollution). This creates free radicals (oxidative stress), which break down cell material and cause inflammation. The suspicion of this correlation is reinforced by the fact that there is a high incidence of melasma in heavily air-polluted countries like India and China [150]. Air pollution is a mixture of particles in gases (e.g., ozone, carbon monoxide, sulphur oxides, nitrogen oxides), organic compounds (from burning garbage, coal, etc. and excretions of bacteria) and metals (e.g., vanadium, nickel and manganese), which can be present indoors and outdoors. When inhaled, swallowed, or even absorbed through the skin, all of these particles alert the immune system and cause inflammation and imbalances in our bodies. We know that melasma is linked to inflammation and oxidative stress and that chemicals can disrupt the endocrine system.

There is emerging evidence that air pollution is a chronic source of inflammatory conditions related to the nervous system (caused by reactive oxygen species (ROS)) [151][152]. An article published in the *Journal of Toxicology and Environmental Health* in 2009 states that air pollution may rank as the most prevalent source of environmentally induced inflammation and oxidative stress [153]. Diesel exhaust particles (DEP), for example, which are common compounds in our outdoor air, are proven to generate free radicals, induce inflammatory responses (cytokines TNF-α and IL-6 and neuropeptide NGF) and stimulate the release of VEGF [34][154].

VEGF, also called vascular endothelial growth factor, is a signalling protein and the factor that drives the new formation of blood vessels. Increased blood vessel formation is a typical reaction of tissues when oxygen is low and is also found in the skin of melasma patients. In a Korean study, skin samples of 50 women with melasma showed an increased number of blood vessels, vessel size, vessel density and elevated VEGF levels in pigmented lesions [155].

The body wants to create more blood vessels in a state of low oxygen because oxygen is carried via blood through the blood vessels. More blood vessels mean a better oxygen supply. The medical term for insufficient oxygen flow to the body tissues is hypoxia, which is another rabbit hole that we will come to shortly and brings us back full circle to facts we have discussed in earlier chapters. The overlap of inflammation, increased blood vessel formation and oxidative stress with melasma and air pollution indicates that the links must be more than just serendipitous.

HYPOXIA AND MELASMA

Can cause:

- oxidative stress

- increase in the number of blood vessels

- overactivity of the immune system and inflammation

Hypoxia alerts your immune system because low oxygen levels bring your body to a dangerous state. We cannot survive without quality and consistent oxygen supply. It is known that cells release the cytokine SCF and the signalling protein VEGF when oxygen levels are low [156]. Additionally, hypoxic states lead to oxidative stress. Deviations in oxygen levels in tissues, whether above or below normal, lead to a loss of electrons in molecules, making them reactive and turning them into free radicals [157][158]. To shock you more, the effects of skin hypoxia can even favour genes that promote melanoma development [159].

BELOW ARE THREE POSSIBLE SCENARIOS IN THE SKIN WHEN OXYGEN IS LOW:

Decreased oxygen » immune system activation » cytokine release with inflammation » pigmentation

Decreased oxygen » more blood vessels » increased oxygen supply to melasma lesions » maintenance of hyperpigmentation

Decreased oxygen » free radical formation » oxidative stress » breakdown of cell material such as cell membrane lipids

But air pollution is not the only problem that can lead to hypoxic states.

According to the Mayo Clinic, three main factors are needed to ensure sufficient oxygen levels in blood and other tissues [160]:

1. Oxygen in the Air

There must be enough oxygen in the air you are breathing. Compromised oxygen in the air is a real environmental issue. According to the National Oceanic and Atmospheric Administration (NOAA) of the United States, it is estimated that $50 - 80\%$ of the oxygen production on Earth comes from the oceans [161]. In particular, plants and bacteria produce most of the oceanic oxygen. The NOAA states that decreased oxygen levels in the oceans "occur most often, however, as a consequence of human-induced factors, especially nutrient pollution from agricultural runoff, fossil-fuel burning and wastewater effluent" [161].

2. Your Breathing

Your lungs must be able to inhale oxygen and exhale carbon dioxide, which is reflected in the way you breathe. Insufficient breathing techniques such as through the mouth, overbreathing and shallow breathing affect your oxygen levels. If carbon dioxide (CO_2) is too low, your red blood cells cannot release oxygen, which causes chronic stress.

3. Blood Circulation

Your bloodstream must be able to circulate blood to your lungs, uptake the oxygen and carry it throughout your body.

Low iron levels are another possible reason for low oxygen, as iron helps to transport oxygen in the blood. About 70% of your body's iron is found in a protein of your red blood cells called haemoglobin. Haemoglobin is essential for transferring oxygen in your blood from the lungs to the tissues. However, supplementing with iron is not necessarily the answer. Furthermore, many heavy metals compete with each other. High copper levels often lead to low iron levels, which we explore in the chapter "Metals".

ARTIFICIAL LIGHT AND LACK OF NATURAL LIGHT AND VITAMIN D

Can cause:

- hyperpigmentation by blue light directly

- shutting down of mitochondria » oxidative stress by blue light

- disruption of the endocrine system by disrupting the circadian rhythm by artificial light

- radiation burns and inflammation by certain types of light

First of all, the sun is your friend, not your foe. Sufficient sunlight is crucial for health and well-being, as our bodies have evolved in synchronicity with the sun. Without the sun, there would be no life. The function of the endocrine system is largely dependent on the spectrum of natural sunlight, as it is one of the major stimuli for hormone production. Our modern lifestyles are shielding us more and more from the natural rays and exposing us to more artificial light than ever before since the invention of the light bulb.

Artificial light is a stressor that can disrupt our circadian rhythm with negative effects on our endocrine system, well-being and skin health. Stress hormones, for example, should naturally be high at daytime and low at night. Artificial light can mess with that natural balance and leave you with high cortisol when you should be winding down. Also, when you are exposed to bright artificial light after sunset, you suppress the action of melatonin, your sleep hormone, sex hormone regulator and also the most potent self-produced antioxidant.

Estrogen production is tightly linked to the circadian rhythm and the action of melatonin. Let me explain the melatonin and estrogen connection in the following passage (also see "How Estrogen is Made in the Body"). When you are outside, sunlight is transferred through the eyes to the hypothalamus in your brain and then to the small pine cone-shaped pineal gland. From there a cascade of chemical actions is set off to stimulate the wake and happy hormone serotonin in the morning. Serotonin is converted into melatonin at night. Therefore, serotonin levels are directly correlated to the amount of sunlight available (= length of day) and directly linked to melatonin levels and sex hormone levels. Longer days mean more sunlight, more serotonin, lower melatonin levels and higher levels of sex hormones. Shorter days mean less sunlight, lower levels of serotonin, higher levels of melatonin and lower levels of sex hormones [162].

This physiology has to do with the fact that nature wants you to be more reproductive when there is more sun because of a better food supply which favours the survival of your offspring. This is how we evolved naturally. In the past, the presence and absence of natural light have determined our life and biology. Nowadays, it is artificial light that determines our wake and sleep cycles. The problem with this is that artificial light bulbs are not emitting the natural spectrum and are also not used during regular day hours but specifically when it is dark outside. We can imagine this can create confusion in our physiology, despite the practical advantages. Low levels of artificial light with an exposure time of only one hour already affect melatonin levels [163][164]. Melatonin levels affect estrogen levels, which we know impacts melasma.

Artificial light, especially blue light, keeps melatonin levels low because the light tells your brain that it is not sleeping time yet. Melatonin impacts estrogen levels because of an enzyme called aromatase. Aromatase converts steroid hormones into estrogen. The lower the melatonin, the higher the aromatase, and the higher the estrogen (artificial light at night » low melatonin » high aromatase » high estrogen) [165].

The correlation between aromatase, melatonin and estrogen is well known in the research and treatment of estrogen-related cancers. Estrogen lowering medications utilised in breast cancer treatment are often aromatase inhibitors. Breast cancer research has picked up on the estrogen and aromatase suppressing effects of melatonin on breast cancer cells [166]. A large survey on shift working women was conducted over several years. A large number of night shift workers have developed endometrial cancer, which the researchers attributed to the low melatonin levels of the women [167].

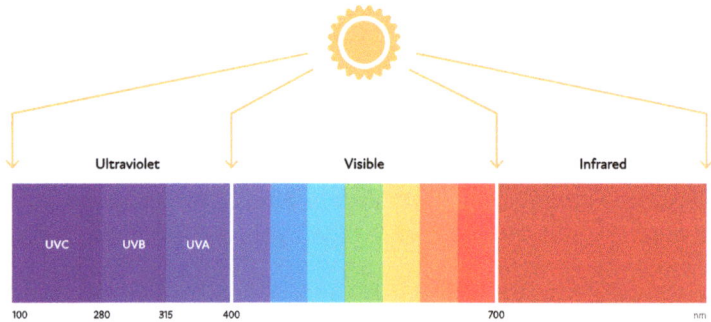

Image 15: The visible light spectrum (Credit: Ansatasia Usenko).

COLOUR	WAVELENGTH
Red	700–635 nm
Orange	635–590 nm
Yellow	590–560 nm
Green	560–520 nm
Cyan	520–490 nm
Blue	490–450 nm
Violet	490–450 nm

Table 10: The wavelengths of the visible light spectrum.

BLUE LIGHT AND PIGMENTATION

In addition to the disrupting effects of artificial light on the endocrine system, there is also a risk of hyperpigmentation from artificial light (even in absence of UV light). Twenty subjects with skin type IV–VI were exposed to two different light sources. One source emitted the entire visible light spectrum ranging from 400–700 nm, the other source was UVA light ranging from 315–400 nm. Surprisingly, visible light in the range between 400 and 700 nm induced darker and more sustained pigmentation compared to the pigmentation induced by UVA [168].

Another research team has assessed the pigmenting effects of visible light on skin explants of human volunteers and found that seven days of light exposure was enough to cause visible brown marks. Those effects were especially apparent in naturally darker skin types [169]. A study from 1988 reported that exposure to an artificial light source with the range of 400–700 nm (entire visible light spectrum) induced not only immediate and lasting skin pigmentation but also inflammation [170].

Another study compared the pigmenting effects of blue-violet, red light and UVB light on human subjects with skin types III–IV. Blue-violet light (415 nm) was found to induce the most pronounced and longest-lasting pigmentation compared to red light (630 nm) and UVB [171]. Blue light is part of the natural spectrum with benefits like increased activity and daytime alertness. Prolonged use of blue light after daylight hours can give us blue light overexposure with effects of low melatonin, mitochondrial shutdown, oxidative stress, skin aging and hyperpigmentation.

We know that when we stay in the sun for too long, we get a burn, which is inflammation that causes oxidative stress as a consequence. But are we aware that working a full day in artificially lit offices and stores can also cause oxidative stress? Several studies confirmed that oxidative stress can be produced in human skin when exposed to artificial light sources in the visible light spectrum with unexpectedly strong effects on the formation of free radicals [172][173].

UV RADIATION

UV radiation (UVA, UVB, UVC light) is the most acknowledged culprit for hyperpigmentation. A large number of studies provide evidence that excess UV radiation has harmful effects like sunburn, oxidative stress and even skin cancer. UV stands for ultraviolet and is part of the non-visible spectrum of light emitted by the sun with a wavelength between 100–400 nm.

UV light is essential for life on earth. We humans possess natural protection against UV radiation, which is our melanin. If the amount of UV radiation exceeds the protective capacity of our melanin content, the skin experiences stress. As a result, our immune system is alerted, and inflammation occurs in the form of sunburn as a mechanism to regain homeostasis and repair the damage. Often after the damage, the skin turns brown. But if certain toxic substances (e.g., medications and metals) are stored in the skin and those intoxicated skin cells are exposed to sunlight, skin cells will activate their protective mechanism (melanin production) earlier and more intensely than usual.

Workers who spend time outside and are exposed to chemicals and pollution, such as farmers and construction workers, and cannot protect themselves from peak UV levels, represent a serious risk group. But what about the people who work indoors? We already have discussed the effects of indoor light in the visible spectrum, but you may not have thought about UV radiation from artificial light sources. UV has the property of exciting fluorescence in materials, which is utilised to produce artificial lighting. Therefore, even indoor light emits some UV light and not just in the range of UVA (315–400 nm) and UVB (280–315 nm), but also the most hazardous UVC rays (100–280 nm). Ultraviolet-emitting light sources used in day-to-day situations include mercury vapor lamps, LED and fluorescent lamps.

THE DANGERS OF UVC

The wavelength of UVC radiation ranges between 100–280 nm and is usually not reaching us on Earth as it is absorbed by the ozone layer. Within the entire spectrum of UV light, UVC has the highest energy and the highest effects in damaging the skin, whilst evoking a stress response [174]. UVC can cause severe burns on the skin and eyes if we come in contact with it. Lamps with a strong UVC emission are utilised in labs to kill microorganisms but usually do not pose any risk to humans due to standard safety measures [175][176].

What we might not be aware of is that commonly used light bulbs, such as compact fluorescent light bulbs (CFL-energy-saving bulbs) emit UVC too. A research team from Stony Brook University in New York found that CFL bulbs emit high levels of UVA and UVC. Exposure of the skin to the light caused significant damage to keratinocytes and fibroblasts and increased oxidative stress. Even though the protective coating of the bulbs should filter the harmful rays, the researchers suspected cracks in the phosphor coating to be responsible for the leakage [177][178]. The same applies to modern LED lights. If the phosphor coating is cracked, UV light will leak [179][180].

Even low UVC emissions can become a problem for people who are exposed to those light sources for long periods of time with negative impacts on their skin and eye health. Especially if the danger is not known and protective measures are not taken. This long-term and accumulated exposure to bright fluorescent light applies especially to occupations like surgeons, nurses and dentists. CFL and mercury vapor light bulbs are slowly banned by certain countries (EU in 2015, US in 2022) but are still not completely removed from our environments.

Another factor to consider regarding UV light is the emission through the window glass of cars and buildings. Window glass blocks most of the UVB that causes sunburn and melanoma but does not filter UVA light as efficiently [181]. UVA is a type of radiation that penetrates deep into the dermis and is known to cause skin aging. The problem with the blocking of UVB through glass is that we are not developing melanin appropriately to shield from UVA rays and also do not have a chance to synthesise vitamin D. As a result, we have ongoing UVA entering our skin into the dermal layer without the natural shielding that would usually occur in natural sunlight.

As we have discussed, fibroblasts are involved in the development of melasma due to their cross-talk with melanocytes and keratinocytes. Because fibroblasts sit in the dermis, it is likely that unfiltered UVA through window glass plays a particular role in the dysfunction of skin pigmentation. Ordinary window glass with a thickness of 4mm can still let 70% of UVA light through (the thicker the glass, the better the UVA absorption) [182]. The UVA absorption in car windows is fairly strong with 96% blockage through front windows but is weaker in the side windows with about 71% blockage. The front window blockage is relatively consistent across different car models and brands but varies greatly in the blockage capacity of side windows [183].

THE ROLE OF VITAMIN D IN MELASMA
The potential risk is:

• a weakened immune system when vitamin D is low

Vitamin D is one of the vital micronutrients humans can produce with sufficient sun exposure and calcium uptake. It is made from cholesterol with the help of photochemical processes after the skin is exposed to UVB sunlight. Vitamin D is not just critical for bone health but also crucial for our immune system and our mood. A study conducted in India found that melasma patients were twice as likely to be insufficient in vitamin D compared to the melasma-free control group. Insufficient levels are quantified as less than 12ng/ml, whereas a normal value is above 20ng/ml [184].

In a Romanian study, all of the 25 female melasma patients enrolled were deficient in vitamin D with an average of 8ng/ml in their blood (the melasma-free control group had an average of 19ng/ml) [185]. It is not clear if low vitamin D directly impacts melasma development or if the low levels result from deficient sun exposure due to a fear of exacerbating pigmentation. Vitamin D deficiency is not a desirable state to be in for immunity and health. In fact, this vitamin has anti-tumour effects [2].

We know that melasma typically appears in people with darker skin. The darker the skin, the more sun exposure people need to have in order to maintain sufficient vitamin D levels. This is because people with darker skin have fewer vitamin D receptors [186]. If you avoid the sun or you apply sunscreen at all times because you are scared to worsen melasma, you set yourself up for low vitamin D. It is recommended to opt for the "do-it-yourself" option of getting out and bathing yourself in the natural sunlight, rather than getting a vitamin D supplement, as the synthetic versions are not as available to the body as the natural and active form (vitamin D3). Considering that we are exposed to so many modern environmental stressors, we require a healthy and supported immune system more than ever. Therefore, we cannot deprive our bodies of this natural and vital nutrient. We can be sun smart and use UV exposure at the right time and to our advantage. You will find smart sunbathing solutions in Part IV.

A REMARK TO ARTIFICIAL LIGHT, NATURAL LIGHT AND VITAMIN D

The message I would like to convey is that we should not demonise the sun but become more aware of circumstances that affect UV exposure and our exposure to artificial light sources. In order to stay healthy, we need to get closer to natural rhythms once again. If we remain terrified of natural sunlight, we deprive ourselves of vitamin D and compromise our immune system.

As an example, in Australia, due to the high incidence of skin cancers, people are very diligent in using sunscreen. Many of my clients had reported to me that they had deficient vitamin D levels when they got their blood checked. It is quite astonishing that there are vitamin D deficient people in a country with so much available sunshine. This exposes the ramifications of fearmongering in regards to sun exposure combined with a lack of valuable and true information. We need better education on how to sunbathe safely without getting burned.

Please see "Sunbathing" in Part IV.

Book recommendation:

"Light in Medicine" by Jacob Lieberman

HEAVY METALS

Can cause:

- oxidative stress » lipid peroxidation [187]

- endocrine system disruption

- inflammation

Metals in tissues have binding properties to melanin, which means that they can hold onto the pigment. Furthermore, melanin acts as a fast ion exchanger for metals, which means with an increased level of metals, there is likely to be more melanin to turn over metals faster. The main pathways of exposure are inhalation, ingestion and skin contact. While some metals are vital to our health, some metals do not belong in our bodies and have detrimental effects. Furthermore, metals often compete with other nutrients, which can negatively affect the endocrine and immune systems.

Maintaining metal homeostasis and the right ratio between metals and minerals are crucial for many different enzymatic activities, cell functions and cell survival.

MERCURY

Can cause:

- oxidative stress

- inflammation

- endocrine system disruption (especially for the thyroid and ovaries)

Mercury is a metal with no nutritional value to the human body but is commonly ingested due to water and seafood contamination. It has a significant and even toxic impact on biological functions in the human body. It is used in batteries, lamps, thermostats, as an antifungal agent in wood processing, preservative for pharmaceutical products, pesticides, fossil fuel combustion from coal and in amalgam fillings. Fortunately, its use was reduced in the 80s and 90s due to federal bans. But because of the heavy use in the past and the pollution from industrial use to this day, mercury exposure is an ongoing event. The main sources of mercury toxicity are fish and dental fillings with amalgam (amalgam fillings contain 50% of mercury [188]). Mercury gets into the water naturally from the Earth's surface and through human pollution into the oceans. It then travels up the food chain from algae to fish to humans eventually [189][190]. Other sources are light bulbs containing mercury, such as mercury vapor lamps and compact fluorescent lamps (CFLs). Breakage in mercury lamps and improper disposal contaminate our environment. It is estimated that about half of the mercury lamps are not appropriately recycled and go into landfills, where they poison our soil, food and water [190].

Due to its oil solubility, mercury can travel rapidly through cell membranes and once inside the cell, it is highly reactive and causes oxidative stress, which then causes inflammation. While there is no direct research on melasma and mercury, a case report mentions skin hyperpigmentation in a woman who has used mercury-contaminated herbal medicines [191]. Mercury can indirectly affect skin pigmentation due to its disrupting effects on the endocrine system. It is found to accumulate in organs like the kidneys, liver and neural tissue, as well as in the pituitary gland, thyroid and ovaries [192][193][194][195][196][197] [198]. Women who had amalgam fillings were asked in a trial to undergo the "chewing gum" test to evaluate their mercury excretion from chewing gum. The results showed that women with hormonal imbalances had the highest secretions of mercury [199].

A study on rats showed that exposure to mercury vapor changed their menstrual cycle [200]. Those changes could be a consequence of the effects mercury has on the reproductive hormones FSH and LH in the pituitary gland (mercury travels easily to the brain) [201]. A survey of 400 dental assistants revealed that those who prepared 30 or more amalgam fillings per week were less fertile than those not exposed to amalgam [202]. Mercury is considered the most toxic heavy metal, and any exposure should be avoided.

COPPER

Can cause:

- increased tyrosinase activity

- inhibition of estrogen clearance

- oxidative stress

Copper is a mineral that is crucial for our vitality and is ingested as a nutrient within our food. Copper can act both as an antioxidant and a pro-oxidant. As an antioxidant, copper neutralises free radicals and can reduce cell damage.

When copper acts as a pro-oxidant, it promotes oxidative stress and can lead to cell, tissue and organ damage, as well as hyperpigmentation. It does not require a big deviation in copper levels to have either toxic or health promoting levels, therefore, copper levels should be well balanced [203]. Copper in excess has a high affinity to store in the liver. Wilson's disease is a genetic dysfunction where the liver cannot metabolise copper properly (the consequence is a copper build-up), and a typical symptom is hyperpigmentation [204].

The reason why copper drives pigmentation is because of the impact it has on the enzyme tyrosinase. Every metal that is a nutrient to the body has a corresponding coenzyme as a catalyst to ensure certain cell functions. Copper needs the enzyme tyrosinase to induce its catalytic effects. In the pigmentation process, this effect is the quick conversion of DOPA (the melanin precursor) into melanin. This means if you have elevated copper levels in your blood or other tissues, you likely have increased tyrosinase activity and subsequently increased melanin formation and hyperpigmentation as a result.

Tyrosinase is just one of the three enzymes involved in the pigmentation process of mammalian skin and it is the most researched one [203]. This enzyme is overactive in most conditions that involve hyperpigmentation, including melasma. Interestingly, the chelation of copper had positive effects on skin pigmentation in a trial that involved patients who developed pigmentation from chlorpromazine use (see chapter "Medication"). The drug did not cause an increase in copper levels itself (at least not reported), but the doctors assumed that copper chelation inactivates tyrosinase and therefore lightens the skin pigmentation [139].

The Indian Journal of Dermatology published an article in 1978 about copper levels in patients with different hyperpigmentary disorders. They found that all patients with hyperpigmentation, including melasma, had significantly higher levels of copper (and copper-binding protein caeruloplasmin) than the control group [205].

Copper tends to be reactive and forms the free radicals superoxide and hydroxyl, leading to oxidative stress [206]. Furthermore, copper affects estrogen and nutrient levels. An excess of copper can lead to high estrogen, low zinc and low iron levels [207]. So, if elevated copper keeps iron levels low, could this decrease oxygen levels and be another explanation for why we find more blood vessels around melasma lesions?

Copper toxicity is unlikely to happen due to eating food that contains copper.

Also, foods rich in copper naturally contain enough zinc to keep a healthy balance. The reason for excess copper can be copper pipes, copper intra-uterine devices (copper IUD – a contraceptive that disturbs the natural hormone cycle), birth control pills, pesticides and medications. I have had several clients with melasma who had a copper IUD.

Read on to find solutions to rid your body of excess copper in Part IV.

NICKEL

Potential risk:

- binding to melanin

When nickel is absorbed in the body and coexists with the chemical compound zinc pyrithione, it forms a complex that can penetrate the cell membranes and binds to pigmented tissues [208].

We are commonly exposed to nickel as it is used in faucets, cookware, jewellery and coins. Unfortunately, water is contaminated with nickel through mining waste. Zinc pyrithione is a chemical compound that has antifungal and antibacterial properties. It is used in antifungal medications, clothing to prevent microbial growth and paint to prevent fungi growth. Because of its antifungal action, it is commonly added to shampoos to treat dandruff.

LEAD

Can cause:

- disruption of the endocrine system

- oxidative stress

- disturbance in the vitamin D metabolism

Lead has no direct effects on hyperpigmentation, but lead toxicity and exposure need adequate attention as it impacts endocrine health, causes oxidative stress and even disturbs vitamin D metabolism. Our environment is contaminated with lead due to fossil fuels, mining and manufacturing. The use of this metal in paint, ceramic, medications and cosmetics are a thing of the past, but lead is still used in pigments and batteries. In the USA alone, 1.52 million tons of lead were utilised in various industries in 2004. 82% of the lead went into battery production [209]. You can imagine how improper battery disposal contaminates our soil and food. Chocolate and coffee commonly contain very high lead levels

[210]. Another common lead source is red lipstick. It is worth it to check chocolate and coffee brands for lead testing. Many companies are conscious of toxicities and test their products. And believe it or not, lead is even found in toilet paper [211]. The contamination of our environment with this toxic metal is omnipresent. Adults absorb 35–50% of lead through drinking water, where it travels through the bloodstream and eventually gets stored in the organs and disrupt the nervous and endocrine system [206]. Lead causes an increase in progesterone levels in women [212] and a decrease in thyroxine levels in male car mechanics [213]. Lead exposure increases lipid peroxidation in workers with high and low lead exposure [214].

A REMARK TO PART III

So far, all the information I have given might be pretty heavy to digest if all this is new to you. My intention is not to make you anxious about risks but to educate you so you can make informed choices. It is my hope that all of us wake up to the fact that it is our collective behaviour and the consequences of this behaviour that are the number one culprits for chronic illness in our society. We need to make lifestyle changes in our daily habits that heal our environment if we want to heal ourselves.

The skin has a significant role in ensuring the body's homeostasis. Environmental toxins absorbed through the skin, inhaled and ingested must be taken seriously as true threats to skin and body health. The increase of the chronic skin condition melasma more likely points to impact factors of the modern world rather than the natural sun. The skin is our gatekeeper; if the skin flares up with chronic blemishes and brown spots, we are being asked by our body to be heard, seen and to investigate what is wrong. The skin is the interface between the inner and outer environment. It is not just regulating itself in response to the inner and outer environment but also reflects these imbalances visibly to the outside. In simpler words, the skin is a reflection of our health. That is why we find smooth and blemish-free skin so attractive. If the skin does not look healthy, we need to start from the inside to fix that. Inner health should be the main focus. We can support skin health by applying potions from nature's medicine cabinet, such as herbs and plant tinctures, but we should not rely on topical treatments alone.

I hope the previous chapters have widened your horizon to the spectrum of skin physiology and health. The spectrum of factors that cause melasma goes far beyond the impact of UV light. The sun should not be demonised as a threat but acknowledged as a healing gift if consumed appropriately. Our daily sun exposure has decreased; in fact, we spend more time indoors than ever. On the other hand, our exposure to emotional stress and toxins due to our disconnection from traditional ways of living, busy lifestyles and industrialisation have increased.

The common assumption in the beauty industry is that melasma is a problem that originates in the melanocytes and therefore is a skin disorder of the epidermal layer. Peels and lasers that reach into the epidermal layer are therefore widely used to treat melasma by beauty therapists, cosmetic nurses and dermatologists, but oftentimes cause inflammation that can exacerbate melasma. Furthermore, some peels and laser treatments used for rejuvenation trigger damage deep in the dermal layers and can create more pigmentation.

PART IV.

HOLISTIC TREATMENT SOLUTIONS

"When a flower doesn't bloom,
you fix the environment in which
it grows, not the flower."

Alexander Den Heijer

The overall goal in treating melasma and healing the skin is to rebalance the body systems (nervous, endocrine and immune systems) and subsequently achieve an optimised equilibrium of body, mind and spirit. This chapter will provide holistic solutions that will tackle the root cause of melasma and provide a true chance to heal from the inside out.

The suggested solutions will help you rebalance your nervous, endocrine and immune systems and naturally reduce oxidative stress and inflammation. As a result, you will not only look good but also feel great. I beg you to be patient with your healing process and to give your body months and maybe even years to improve. The first step in the healing approach offered in this book is the analysis of the possible imbalance; step two discusses the detox process; and step three covers the healing methods.

The detox solutions in this chapter will help to clear toxins from your tissues. The process of detoxing is a little bit like treating a stain on your clothes. The first idea that would probably come to your mind is to remove the stain by rinsing the piece and cleansing it, instead of just dabbing on something to dissolve it. The same principle applies to our bodies. The removal of the culprit is the first step to healing.

The healing and nourishing solutions will further allow the rebalancing and maintenance of your body's homeostasis. The solutions require living a healthy lifestyle, which may demand changes and efforts in your life but will ensure long-lasting results.

IDENTIFICATION AND TESTING FOR IMBALANCES

SELF-ENQUIRY

Self-enquiry about symptoms and history can be very helpful in identifying possible issues, especially if you know what to ask. You can find a questionnaire in the appendix for a deep dive. This should provide guidance on where to start. If you identify toxins in your daily life, the first step is to eliminate those. If you suspect that you have a hormone imbalance, I recommend investing in a hormone test. If you realise that you have significant stressors in your life, now is a good time to start reducing those however possible.

An exercise for self-enquiry could also go as follows if you do not want to answer the questionnaire: Sit in silence and ask yourself what factors in your life could cause these imbalances. Where is your body, mind and spirit not looked after or aligned? Let the answers come to you. Take your time with this; write the answers down. Below are some examples of how to start self-enquiry.

BODY	MIND	SPIRIT
Do I get enough sunlight?	What are my daily thoughts?	Am I receiving enough love?
Do I eat a healthy and diverse diet?	Do I feel overwhelmed by my work load?	Am I trusting?
Do I move enough?	What are stressors in my life?	Do I love myself?
How is my breathing?	Do I have enough downtime?	Have I dealt with my traumas?
Do I get enough rest and sleep?	What are my coping mechanisms?	Do I have faith that there is something bigger that holds and supports me?

Table 11: Examples of questions for self-enquiry

HORMONE TESTING

Before we go into any treatment suggestions or customised protocols to rebalance your endocrine system, it is best to identify possible imbalances first to ensure the best outcome. A good start is to answer the questionnaires for yourself. Then, if you have suspicions about hormone imbalances or are experiencing obvious symptoms, the next step could be to see a doctor to identify imbalances via a blood or urine test. An alternative is to order lab tests yourself. If you order tests from a laboratory, you need to have your blood taken by a doctor or nurse; then, they send it to the lab for analysis.

The DUTCH test (dried urine test) provides a comprehensive and very detailed analysis of your hormone levels. It gives more in-depth information than a standard blood serum test. The advantage of DUTCH testing is that you and your practitioner can much better identify what specific hormone is elevated or decreased, why this is the case and if there are elimination pathways blocked. DUTCH tests are pricier than blood serum tests but are undoubtedly worth it. Dr. Carrie Jones is a renowned doctor in Integrative and Functional Medicine who specialises in this particular test (https://dutchtest.com/author/carrie-jones-nd-mph).

Once you have the test results, a doctor of Integrative, Naturopathic or Chinese Medicine you trust can help you create a customised and root cause based treatment. Treating mild endocrine imbalances that are not life-threatening does not require prescription drugs. I can vouch for that from my own experience. Your body can heal itself if you provide the right environment. Everyone's health improves significantly and often quickly once the culprits we have discussed in Part III are eliminated from your system. But please remember, true healing and reversing conditions still require patience. More on how to do that soon.

GUT MICROBIOME TESTING

A comprehensive gut microbiome test can identify imbalances and which foods contribute to your health or which you should avoid.

Gut microbiome testing providers: www.viome.com

DNA ANALYSIS

Modern DNA testing can provide a practical insight into food sensitivities, which can help you to avoid inflammation caused by the food you eat or supplements you take. Lowering inflammation is a critical part of healing melasma.

DNA testing providers: www.thednacompany.com

HEAVY METAL TESTING

There are different ways to find out if you have metal toxicity. You can get your blood, hair, or urine tested. The only downside with blood or urine testing is that only circulating metal ions from recent intake or metal that is in the process of being chelated from tissues can be detected. If you have metals stored in tissues, organs or glands, a blood test or urine test will not be able to give insight.

As an alternative to blood, hair and urine testing, I can recommend a quantum resonance screening. I would have never known about lead in my thyroid without this screening. About ten years ago, I had blood taken and was diagnosed with an underactive thyroid, but I rejected the medication. I had typical symptoms like low energy, cold hands and feet. Then, I got a recommendation from a friend to do a quantum resonance screening and did it just for fun. I sat at the practitioner's office with a helmet on my head attached to a computer and a software program. Interestingly, the lead in my thyroid was the most distinctive issue and possibly the reason for my imbalanced thyroid levels from years ago. I got a chelating homeopathic blend prescribed and felt improvements in my well-being within six weeks. A quantum resonance screening is a modern diagnostic tool that picks up on changes in the frequencies of cells in your body and can detect the buildup of stored metals.

Quantum resonance device for screening: https://nls-diagnostic.com

Heavy metal hair test: www.upgradedformulas.com

MOLD TESTING

If you had water damage in the house and believe you have mold in your home, you can find companies in your area via web search that help you test and treat your home for mold.

Testing for mold in your body is more challenging and maybe not as crucial as a hormone test. Following a mold detox protocol is not dangerous and is beneficial for overall detox. But if you want to be certain whether you have toxicity from mold, you can test for antibodies (IgG–Immunoglobulin G) in your blood to see if your immune system shows typical signs of mold exposure or get a mycotoxin urine test.

DETOX

DETOX YOUR HOUSEHOLD AND COSMETIC SHELF

Benefits:

- supports and rebalances the endocrine system

- de-stresses the immune system

- reduces inflammation

- reduces oxidative stress

Get rid of all toxic personal care, and cleaning products, textiles and toxic cookware. Living a toxin-free life will be a game-changer for optimised physical health. Many cosmetic and household products contain endocrine disruptors, pesticides and heavy metals.

What you can do:

- Reduce plastic use to reduce BPA and phthalate exposure.

- Drink spring water or filtered water to avoid metal toxicity.

- Eat organic as much as possible to avoid ingesting pesticides.

- Invest in high-quality textiles like clothing, bed linen, towels, etc., to avoid skin contact and respiratory system ingestion of chemicals.

- No fake jewellery due to the high chance of allergic reactions; wearing real gold and silver even has health benefits.

- Carpets, furniture and mattresses also often contain toxins; research before buying new ones.

- Use organic and toxin-free cosmetics, make-up, nail polish, hair products and toothpaste.

- Use toxin-free cleaning products (also laundry and dish detergent). Essential oils, baking soda, vinegar and citric acid are great cleaning alternatives.

- Invest in good cookware (ceramic and cast iron).

- Avoid buying anything that smells suspiciously chemically (with a pungent scent).

- If you see mold on your furniture, wipe the items down with white vinegar (add clove essential oil if you have it). Place items outside in the sun for a few hours. Sunlight is a great pathogen killer.

Check out:

- www.ewg.org » Environmental Working Group, for more information and solutions, also available as an app

- www.ecospecifier.com.au » huge database for safe consumer products

DETOX YOUR BODY

SWEATING

Benefits

- helps to eliminate toxins

- increases mitochondrial health

- decreases oxidative stress

1. Movement and Exercising

   High-intensity workouts, hot yoga, dancing and aerobics are a few examples.

2. Sauna

   Sweating is good for you and is a natural way to eliminate toxins from the body. Because of the potentially unpleasant smell, we try to inhibit sweating as much as possible. But deodorant can block the pathways that allow toxins to exit the body via sweat glands. This can lead to a toxic overload in your body and skin problems like severe acne. If you find that your armpits smell bad, even if you had a shower recently, it can be a sign of accumulated toxins in your body. Apply a clay mask (bentonite is best) on your armpits for 10–20 minutes to detox the area; you will feel fresh afterwards. Keeping the detox pathways in your armpits clean is also beneficial for breast health. For unpleasant smells, you can use a single drop of organic essential oil between your palms and dab it on your armpits as a scented replacement for deodorant.

GET LYMPH MOVING

1. Movement

Your lymph pathways are also one of your elimination systems. Toxins are filtered through your lymph nodes, and movement is the best way to get the lymph flowing. Because your body is smart, your lymph nodes are located in areas where a lot of movement is required, like joints. Rotate your joints, pump your arms, squat, etc. Get creative and have fun with it.

2. Dry Brushing

Before a shower, swim or sauna, brush for 2–10 min in a circular motion towards the heart. Start on the right foot, move up to the hips, then the left foot, and up to the hip again. Then from the right hand up to the shoulders and so on.

3. Cold Shower

A cold shower at the end of each warm shower benefits capillary health and firms the tissues.

4. Massage

Receiving professional lymph drainage is a lovely pampering self-care ritual. Giving yourself a massage with oil gets the lymph flowing as well. Use gentle pressure.

FASTING AND DETOX FROM FOOD ADDITIVES

Benefits:

• de-stresses the immune system

• reduces inflammation

FASTING

Fasting is an ancient purification method that is still practised to this day and a solid pillar of many religions worldwide. With the historical disconnection of the western world from religion and spirituality, the fasting tradition seems to have been lost as well but is making a revival as an alternative healing method. Whether you fast only from certain foods or food altogether for some time, it will benefit your health. Refraining from certain foods that burden your body supports the healing process and can de-stress your immune system. Abstaining from food altogether for a period of time helps your body focus purely on renewal and repair without the need for energy for digestion. Fasting is an accelerator to chelate toxins and can reset your relationship with food and your sense of taste.

Additionally, you start to burn fat after 36 hours of fasting, which is a great way to release toxins that are stored in fat cells. Often, the release of toxins from fat cells can make you feel tired or even unwell for a bit since these toxins are now circulating in your system, ready to be eliminated. If you plan a fast, make sure you do it during a time that allows you to rest.

Fasting has an additional benefit if extended for several days. After five days of fasting, a process called autophagy sets in. It rids the body of damaged cells and proteins and even repairs stem cells. Endogenous antioxidants, like NAD+ and rejuvenating hormones like HGH increase. Blood sugar levels stabilise, which reduces inflammation. Dr. Jason Fung has cured patients with Diabetes II with his water fasting method and describes the process in his book "The Complete Guide to Fasting".

Book recommendation: "The Complete Guide to Fasting" by Dr. Jason Fung

REFRAINING FROM SPECIFIC FOODS AND FOOD ADDITIVES

As much as food can be a healer, food treated with chemicals is toxic. Many nutritionists believe that sensitivities from food are a reaction to pesticides rather than a reaction to the food itself, which is one reason to opt for organic food. Another reason to choose organic food is that the nutrient density is higher. It is known that pesticides change the pH level of the soil to a more acidic pH. For the soil to have optimum levels of minerals in order to pass them onto vegetables and fruits, the pH needs to be alkaline [215]. More minerals in the soil mean more minerals in your food.

The most inflammatory foods to avoid are corn, wheat, sugar and soy as well as food additives that are derived from them. To reduce inflammation, it is best to avoid inflammatory foods altogether for at least four weeks to see if you notice positive changes. That does not mean that these foods are generally bad. Corn, wheat and soy have been important staple foods across different cultures since the beginning of agriculture and were not a problem until modern times.

The problem is that these foods are highly processed, genetically modified and laden with pesticides. To calm your body from inflammation, try to eat only organic fruit and veggies for a month or longer if you can. Then reintroduce wheat, corn and soy (one at a time and only if you want to) in pure, organic and fermented form (such as sourdough and tempeh). Find a table of food additives to avoid during your healing period in the appendix (Table 11).

Also, please avoid drinks like kombucha when you are inflamed. Kombucha is high in histamines and can add to inflammation when your body is already inflamed.

I also recommend reducing or even totally avoiding sugar as it causes inflammation and excess estrogen. Excess sugar is converted to lipids in the liver, leading to decreased sex hormone binding globulin (SHBG) levels. SHBG binds sex hormones, and a decrease in this protein means an increase in estrogen and testosterone [216]. Do not feel reluctant to eat fruit. Fruit is a healer. It is the refined sugars that are too much for the body to process and does not come with all the other nutrients when consumed in sugary foods and drinks.

Also, dairy and gluten can cause inflammation and should be avoided to reduce inflammation levels. According to Dr. Wentz, improvements in her patient's symptoms with Hashimoto's are seen within days when ditching dairy and gluten (Hashimoto's is also connected to low stomach acid and insufficient microbiome) [72].

It seems tedious to check all food labels for those ingredients, but it does not have to be complicated. The easiest method to avoid those additives is to buy and eat only foods with no label (whole and real foods like vegetables, fruits and legumes) or where the label contains a handful of simple and natural ingredients that you can easily identify. Please also keep in mind that a lot of low-quality supplements and protein powders (which can still be expensive) contain these food additives.

This is the detox part of the dietary solution. Find more about nutrition and diet soon under "Heal & Nourish".

DETOX FROM METALS

Benefits:

- supports endocrine health

- reduces oxidative stress

- reduces inflammation

- improves nutrient uptake

During a metal detox protocol, it is important to avoid the reuptake of metals. Otherwise, any detox or chelation treatment is rather pointless. The best avoidance practice is eliminating possible heavy metal sources. This includes avoiding tap water or the removal of the copper IUD if you have one. If you are considering removing your copper IUD, be aware that the removal can release copper into the system. Therefore, binding and chelating copper particles during and after removal should be considered. When copper levels are high, zinc levels are usually low. Zinc is a safe mineral to take as a supplement and can help to balance copper levels. Avoid mercury-laden fish and seafood. Some fish are considered safer than others. Tuna, for example, is more mercury-laden than salmon [217].

Antioxidants like vitamin C, E, melatonin, glutathione, superoxide dismutase, catalase, glutathione peroxidase and glutathione reductase help to chelate and neutralise the effects of metals [218]. We have to get vitamin C and E from our foods, all other components mentioned are made in the body (mainly in the mitochondria). Alpha-lipoic acid is another antioxidant made in the mitochondria, which has chelating properties on metals [219]. You can also find it in broccoli, potatoes and spinach. The binding property of alpha-lipoic acid to metals is accredited to the sulphur atoms. Sulphur is a chelating agent that has gained some attention as a metal chelating solution [220] found in all cruciferous vegetables and garlic. The chelating effects of metals from body-made antioxidants like glutathione, alpha-lipoic acid and melatonin show how important the health of mitochondria and the endocrine system is (melatonin is made in the pineal gland and mitochondria).

Activated charcoal has an excellent chelation property for lead, copper and nickel due to its large absorption surface and ability to hold the weight of metal ions [221][222]. Please choose activated charcoal from a high-quality source. Coconut shell is considered the best source [223]. Some charcoal powders come from burned wood or are contaminated with other substances that can be toxic.

By ingesting detoxifying foods and charcoal or other binders, small molecules that act like magnets circulate via the blood through all your organs and glands and bind metal ions to them.

Additionally, if you avoid heavy metal uptake in the future and consume a good diet, your body will eliminate metals over time by natural cell renewal. The part of your body which takes the longest to renew is your skeleton. It takes about ten years to renew the entire bone structure. Other organs are quicker. The epidermis only takes about a month to renew. It is fantastic to know that with a change of lifestyle and patience, we can renew our entire body.

The chelation of metals can be dangerous if not done correctly, as freed metal ions can go to the brain and cause more damage than good. The safest way to chelate metals is under the guidance of a trained practitioner. But if you follow specific guidelines and are healthy otherwise, do not take medication and feel confident about taking control of your own health, you can certainly do an at-home chelation.

HOW TO DO AN AT-HOME CHELATION:

1. It is important to eat very healthily and to drink a lot of water during the detox process to ensure secretion pathways are open and clear. It is important not to drink alcohol or to use medications that are counterproductive. The liver is one of the most important detox organs, so you do not want to burden the liver with other toxins. Also, eating a fibre-rich diet is essential to transport toxins.

2. Keep up with your daily intake of probiotics for your gut health.

3. Protect your brain by keeping antioxidant levels high. Eat fresh vegetables and fruits (sulphur rich) and improve healthy mitochondrial function by:

   a. Daily exercise.

   b. Fasting periods or intermittent fasting.

   c. Sufficient sunlight at sunrise and sunset for melatonin production. Melatonin is a potent antioxidant made in the pineal gland of the brain and mitochondria.

   d. Enough sleep.

4. Drink activated charcoal after waking (at least 30 min before your first meal). Add a heaping tablespoon to a glass of water. Do this daily for 14 days, then rest for 7–14 days. Repeat the on and off cycle for up to 6 months. There are different protocols and recommendations out there. Do what feels right for you and choose the protocol of your liking by doing some research.

5. Drink only spring or filtered water. Tap water often contains heavy metals.

This method can help to detox from other toxins as well. Charcoal is a toxin binder that has been used in traditional and modern medicine for a long time.

Additionally, we all can contribute to reducing future metal pollution from mercury, lead and other metals by properly recycling batteries and mercury lamps to avoid contamination of soils and water (Please check at your municipal governing body for arrangements of hazardous goods collections.).

DETOX FROM MEDICATIONS

Benefits:

- reduces oxidative stress

- reduces inflammation and de-stresses the immune system

Antibiotics, antidepressants and many other drugs are a blessing in many circumstances and often are life-saving. But remember that the healthier your body is, the less likely you will be in need of medications. Your day-to-day commitment to health is the best medicine. Medications should be a short-term solution to regulate acute issues, but they will not help you to regain true health. After every medication use, there is a chance of residues in the body.

The cleaner your diet, the better you support your body to detox those residues, as your body does not have to deal with additives and toxins from food. After using antibiotics, it is essential to restore gut health with probiotics. Good-quality fermented foods like yoghurt, sauerkraut, tempeh and natto are excellent alternatives to probiotic capsules and a source of living cultures that also have additional nutrient value.

Also, see "Detox from Metals" for a detox protocol.

DETOX FROM RADIATION AND ARTIFICIAL LIGHT

Benefits:

- a balanced endocrine system

- better mitochondrial health

- reduced oxidative stress

WHAT YOU CAN DO TO PROTECT YOURSELF FROM ARTIFICIAL BLUE LIGHT OVERLOAD:

1. Replace bright lighting at home with incandescent light bulbs or blue-light-blocking light bulbs.

2. Choose lower wattage light bulbs.

3. Use candlelight instead of artificial light.

4. Use blue blockers as glasses during screen time.

5. Apply blue light filters on computer and phone screens.

6. Adjust the blue light emission with filter adjustment on your devices.

WHAT YOU CAN DO TO PROTECT YOURSELF FROM RADIO WAVES:

1. Turn your phone to airplane mode if you are not using it and especially if you have it close to your body.

2. Choose hands-free when having phone calls (avoid Bluetooth earphones).

3. Opt for the ethernet cable option for your home internet.

4. When moving to new places, check how close you are to electricity lines and cellular towers.

5. Wear radiation protection clothing.

WHAT YOU CAN DO TO PROTECT YOURSELF FROM SPLIT UV LIGHT AND PEAK HOUR UV:

1. Use car window shields to the sides.

2. Cover up with long clothes and thin natural fabrics during peak hours (loose white linen is best).

3. Wear hats.

4. If you need sunscreen, zinc is the least toxic solution.

5. Try to avoid sitting too close to windows.

RADIATION PROTECTION BRANDS:

Radiasmart (clothing), Leela Quantum Tech (household and clothing), Defender Shield (for devices)

Blue light blocking glasses and light bulbs:

Ra Optics, BLUblox

DETOX FROM AIR POLLUTION
Benefits:

- reduces oxidative stress

- de-stresses the immune system

- reduces inflammation

DETOX OUTDOOR AIR

Everyone can contribute to cleaner outdoor air by becoming more conscious about emission levels in our daily habits. It is our behaviour within our environment that makes us sick and makes us look sick, so it is our behaviour that can make us be well and look well.

1. Choose local. Every product we buy has to travel. We can choose to support local products and thereby reduce travel time and fuel emissions while ensuring freshness.

2. We can reduce emissions from our cars by choosing to walk, bike or

take public transport whenever possible.

3. We can consciously choose to buy from companies that regrow forests or donate to associations that plant trees. Plants absorb carbon dioxide and produce oxygen by photosynthesis. The more plants we grow, the more carbon dioxide we can turn over.

4. Reduce electricity use. The burning of fossil fuels for energy pollutes the air directly and indirectly by acidifying the ocean. Ocean acidification leads to algae death, affecting the oxygen levels in the air.

5. Conscious buying of furniture and other household goods. Checking energy efficiency levels of electronic appliances like washing machines.

6. Support businesses that support the regrowth of forests. Check out rainforest ceramics in Australia. Every pottery piece purchased helps to regrow the rainforest. Richard is the potter and was the man who registered Greenpeace in Australia (rainforestceramics.com).

7. Use less plastic to avoid ocean pollution. A significant amount of ocean pollution is the result of plastic waste from our households. As discussed in Part III, most of our ambivalent oxygen comes from the oceans, and its pollution is a significant factor in the deprivation of oxygen levels.

8. Use fewer chemical fertilisers for your garden and buy organic produce. A considerable amount of chemicals used in agriculture make it to the ocean through waterways, even when the distance to the ocean is far.

9. Do not allow chemicals to go into the sink or toilet. Use toxin-free cleaning products and detergents. Waste water goes through the sewage system into the ocean.

DETOX INDOOR AIR

Air Purifiers and Indoor Plants

An indoor air purifier with a HEPA filter is a great way to help remove airborne toxins in your home. But electrical purifiers have downsides as they emit harmful chemicals, cause noise pollution and use energy. Plants deliver excellent air-purifying properties and look beautiful. The top 12 air-purifying plants are listed below. You need 1 or 2 plants per 9.3 square metres to clean the air.

- Bamboo palm

- Boston fern

- Peace lily

- Mother-in-law's tongue

- Florist's chrysanthemum

- Corn plant

- English ivy

- Spider plant

- Weeping fig

- Chinese evergreen

- Philodendron sp

- Barberton or transvaal daisy, gerbera

Burning organic essential oils like eucalyptus can purify the air in your home and can help with respiratory and sinus health. Generally speaking, the less toxic your home textiles and furniture are, the fewer toxins become volatile and get into your indoor air.

DETOX FROM MOLD

If you have the suspicion that mold toxicity might apply to you due to self-enquiry or if you have the proof from a test result, then this is for you:

1. Get out of the mold exposure.

2. Avoid foods that potentially harbor molds or choose options of a higher quality. Buy from a farmer you trust. Some companies test their products for mycotoxins.

3. Check for water damage when moving into new places.

4. Avoid buying second-hand furniture that is hard to clean (upholstered furniture).

5. Wipe down furniture with a mix of white vinegar and clove essential oil (you can add water for sensitive surfaces 1:1). Place items in the midday sun. If the mold regrows, it is better to dispose of the item.

6. Dehumidifiers in tropical areas can be life-changing.

7. Sweat and ensure healthy bowel function to get rid of internal mold toxicity.

8. Drink bentonite clay (1 tbsp) mixed with water first thing in the morning. Drink a lot of water to avoid constipation. Allow a couple of off days per week.

9. Rebuild your gut microbiome with probiotics, various foods and environments (breathe in different environments from forests to meadows, beaches, etc.).

HEAL AND NOURISH

REDUCING EMOTIONAL AND MENTAL STRESS

Benefits:

- calms the nervous system

- rebalances the endocrine system by reducing the stress response

- reduces inflammation

3 ACTIVE STEPS TO HEAL FROM EMOTIONAL AND MENTAL STRESS:

1. Identify your stressors. When do you get stressed?

2. Think about ways to reduce or eliminate stressors.

E.g., if you notice that you crumble underneath too many responsibilities, are there any options to delegate the workload to people around you? Feeling responsible for too many tasks is a typical disease. Most of us are guilty of that. It is worth it to explore why that is the case. Do we believe that we are the only ones who can accomplish these tasks? Do we feel more worthy if we do it all alone? Are we trying to fill up an account to then be allowed to ask for things we need? It goes deep...but saying no is ok. Do not empty yourself to help and please everyone else before yourself.

3. Find tools that suit your schedule to calm yourself in stressful moments.

E.g., breathing exercises, movement and meditation.

TOOLS FOR STRESS REDUCTION

NOSE BREATHING AND BREATHING TECHNIQUES

One would think there are no instructions needed for proper breathing. We all have done it from the minute we left our mom's belly. However, people seem to be at a loss when remembering what appropriate breathing is. Improper breathing can occur because of a disconnection we have with our bodies or our inherited anatomy or even anatomical changes due to accidents or adaptions. Many among us are mouth breathers, which negatively affects our nervous system. James Nestor has dedicated a whole book to breathing and explains the science behind the ancient wisdom of proper breathing. A wide range of benefits encompasses, regulating the nervous system, a better appearance and improved sleep. The reason why nose breathing is so beneficial is that it allows high levels of nitric oxide from the sinuses to mix with inhaled oxygen. This process helps to kill bacteria and to remove dust, mildew, mold, animal dander, smoke and other irritants from the inhaled air. Mouth breathing on the other hand, can keep the immune system overstimulated, which leads to inflammation.

Additionally, without nitric oxide entering the lungs as a bronchodilator, lower oxygen saturation levels may occur in the blood [224]. Low oxygen saturation, also called hypoxia, is mentioned in Part III "Air Pollution". Slow breaths into your belly with longer exhales than inhales, with five breaths per minute, maintain good blood oxygenation and have instantly calming effects on your nervous system [225]. It is a good practice to pay attention to your breathing all day long and slow down if you catch yourself breathing too fast or not at all. When sudden anxiety hits or a situation makes your heart beat out of control, try this:

Close your right nostril and breathe deeply in and out through your left nostril until you feel calmer. Once calm, breathe through both nostrils again. It helped me so many times when my nervous system was spiralling out of control. When you breathe through your left nostril, you deactivate the sympathetic nervous system while your parasympathetic nervous system is engaged automatically.

Book recommendation: "Breath" by James Nestor

MOVEMENT

Get moving but in a way that serves you, your body, mind and spirit. Listen and trust your intuition. Walk, dance, shake it out, hula hoop, play, go on a trampoline or do yoga.

Muscle tension is a typical sign of stored emotional trauma and stress. There is a technique called "Trauma Release Exercise" (TRE) to release those trauma storages. The exercises are designed to tire out specific muscle groups until you start shaking. If we look at tribes worldwide, dancing used to be a daily practice, and traditional tribal dances involve a lot of shaking. I always think about how ecstatic Tina Turner used to dance and how that must have saved her sanity during decades of physical abuse. When animals are confronted with a threat, they instantly shake and tremble afterwards. We have all seen that with dogs and even with ducks, which flap their wings after a confrontation. Our social norms have forbidden us to exert such behaviours in public to fit in and be accepted.

SEX AS STRESS RELIEVER

Sex is a stress reliever–with yourself, your partner or others. Having an orgasm is an effective stress reliever as it releases the hormones oxytocin and dopamine. Both hormones relieve stress by lowering cortisol levels.

GAINING SPIRITUAL STRENGTH

Whether you follow certain religious beliefs or believe in the spiritual realm without a specific framework, believing in a higher power that supports you through life is a powerful tool, no matter how disastrous the situation you are in. Growing up without religious or spiritual beliefs, I can confirm that faith has been a healer for me and supports me through my daily life to feel safe and sane. For me, connecting to nature, connecting to myself and the spirit realm through meditation has opened up a pathway to spiritual strength.

A great way to strengthen spirituality is with the awareness and training of chakras. Activating and strengthening chakras is a tool taught in ancient Indian yogic traditions. The chakras are also referred to as wheels of light or energy (as in Sanskrit chakra = wheel or disc). There are seven different chakras within the body, which are located along the spine. Each chakra represents different glands, organs, emotions and even colours. Yogi masters and teachers say that when your chakras are vital, you are strong and healthy physically, mentally and spiritually. The efficacy of yoga and meditation, which focuses on the chakras, is proven by the popularity among Western people, who become increasingly disconnected and sick, finding solace in ancient Eastern traditions.

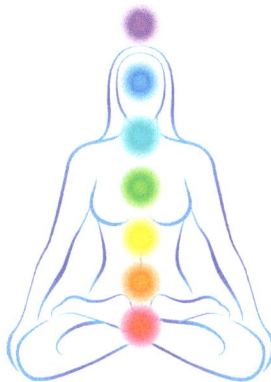

Image16: The chakra system
(Credit: PeterHermesFurian).

One of the most targeted practices to train your chakras is kundalini yoga, brought into our Western world by yogi Bhajan. I would describe kundalini yoga as a mystical form of yoga. The movements, also called kriyas, are performed or held for an extended time and can physically challenge you so much that you enter a different realm mentally and spiritually. You train not only a healthy body but also a strong mind and spirit. The effects are profound and instantly noticeable. Russell Brand, Cindy Crawford, Gabrielle Bernstein and many others are advocates of this life-changing practice.

Benefits of Kundalini Yoga:

- balances the endocrine system and nervous system

- reduces stress

- emotional balance

- detox

- spiritual, mental and physical stamina

Recommendations for teachers who offer online training:

Gurmukh Khalsa, Guru Jagat, Victoria Latham, Kimilla

BUILDING A SUPPORT NETWORK

You do not have to become an extrovert if you are an introvert, but having a support network, like-minded people or even a soul tribe family around you is a powerful stress reducer. It can even be an online community you connect to regularly. The feeling of being connected to others can be very soothing and can help relieve loneliness.

HEALING PAST EMOTIONAL TRAUMA

Some believe that physical disease is caused by emotional and spiritual imbalances and manifests as somatic conditions, even if biological factors do not cause it (e.g., muscle tension or autoimmune disorders). You may have heard of psychosomatic illness. It describes a condition that manifests physically but is caused by psychological stress. Chronic skin conditions belong to those psychosomatic conditions. Research is also acknowledging that emotional trauma can cause autoimmune disease. The work of Dr. Gabor Mate, a physician and expert in emotional trauma healing, focuses on the recovery of our traumatised society. His work has helped thousands of people and will hopefully spread far and wide.

Looking for professional help and opening up to a psychologist with whom we do not have a personal relationship and who does not judge us can bring immense healing. Talking about your story helps your healing process as it allows the mental and physical energy of the event to dissipate over time [112].

DEVELOPING LOVE FOR SELF

When we were emotionally stressed as children, we would usually go to our mothers to soothe us and to calm our nervous system. Research shows that our nervous systems as children are still closely connected to our mothers. This was our first love relationship, and we were emotionally dependent on our mothers and caregivers. In the phase of growing up, we gain more independence from our mothers and tend to redirect the reliance on soothing and nervous system regulation to other people or things, usually romantic partners, substances or material things. Unfortunately, many of us were never taught to build a loving relationship with ourselves to self-regulate.

Self-regulation is a powerful tool to calm your nervous system and rebalance yourself. Being there for ourselves and loving ourselves can heal us in many ways. Saying loving words and thinking loving thoughts to yourself generates electrical impulses in your brain and heart, sending them through your nervous system. These are eventually received as loving frequencies in each of your cells. If your cells vibrate at a loving frequency, you have no other choice but to feel at ease.

An exercise to practice self-love is to activate your heart chakra. Close your eyes, and place your hands on your heart. Breathe in and out through your nose and imagine a green or pink light in your heart centre. With every inhale, the light becomes more extensive and brighter; with every exhale, the loving light permeates through your cells, fills your entire body, and eventually swirls around you. Say wonderful things to yourself that you would tell a person you love dearly. Direct all the love you have for yourself. You might experience a firework of sparks right in your heart centre; you deserve it. Louise Hay was a teacher of self-love who helped millions of people. Her book "You Can Heal Your Life" offers the most amazing and easy-to-apply methods to practice self-love.

Book recommendation: "You Can Heal Your Life" by Louise Hay

FOOD IS A HEALER

"Let food be thy medicine, and let medicine be thy food." – unknown [226]

Benefits:

- heals the endocrine system

- strengthens the immune system

- increases antioxidant levels

- reduces oxidative stress

- improves lipid barrier function

Food is an essential contributor to our physical health. I do not want to make this book about diet and therefore will not go into details about nutrition, but I will give you some advice that is easy to follow and helped me on my healing journey. Nutrient-dense, organic food and spring water help your body to heal by slowly removing toxins from your cells whilst nourishing your body. Foods rich in fibre help your body with the elimination of excess hormones and waste products. Fresh foods also carry life force energy conveyed as frequencies that have healing properties (more about healing frequencies in "Frequency Healing").

Rather than asking ourselves how many calories are in food x, y or z, instead ask how many nutrients can I get from that meal. How can I prepare my food to get maximum nutrient density? What foods in the food court or restaurant menu have the highest nutrient value? The more nutrients you ingest, the better and the faster you are satiated. On my journey, the cleaner my diet became, the more connected I became to my body. The more connected we become to our body, the more we strengthen our natural ability to eat intuitively. A balanced diet with balanced amounts of protein, carbs and fat is better than any trendy diet. Add diversity to your diet. The higher the variety, the more diversity you have in your microbiome. You cannot go wrong with fresh, organic vegetables to reduce inflammation and nourish your body with the nutrients it needs for a well-functioning endocrine system.

Cooking meals from scratch ensures a clean diet. And it does not have to be a complicated meal. When I have little time, I eat plain basmati rice with steamed or fried broccoli and garlic. It sounds boring, but I find it delicious and it is neither expensive nor time consuming. This might sound disappointing, but food is meant to nourish, not to excite our taste buds. Broccoli belongs to the group of cruciferous vegetables together with Brussels sprouts and kale. These are high in fibre and help to open elimination pathways to excrete excess hormones. Beans and legumes are also high in fibre but should be soaked for at least 6 hours to reduce inflammatory histamine levels (then discard the soaking water).

Do not forget herbs and spices like parsley and coriander, which help to chelate heavy metals. Fresh herbs also carry high vibrational energy, whilst turmeric is an anti-inflammatory spice.

Drinking spring water or filtering your water at home with a filtering system limits your heavy metal uptake.

Also, our eating "style" greatly impacts our digestion and nutrient uptake. We need to chew our food properly to make enough stomach acid. The chewing action in your mouth produces acid in your stomach. Low stomach acid is connected to food sensitivity due to a decreased breakdown of food, which causes inflammation. Low stomach acid also promotes the overgrowth of gut bacteria. Digestive enzymes as a supplement can help to break down food if low stomach acid is an issue or if you have eaten food you usually react to.

Book recommendation: "The Beauty Detox Power: Nourish Your Mind and Body for Weight Loss and Discover True Joy" by Kimberly Snyder

TARGETED GUT HEALING AND MICROBIOME RESTORATION

Benefits:

- strengthens the immune system

- reduces inflammation

Maintaining a healthy and balanced gut microbiome is crucial for a strong immune system and for lowering inflammation.

1. Eliminate foods like corn, wheat, dairy, soy and refined sugar (including alcohol) for 4–6 weeks.

2. Restore the gut with probiotics.

3. Help digestion with digestive enzymes.

4. Heal with homemade bone or vegetable broth.

5. You can slowly reintroduce foods, but please choose organic, non-GMO and properly prepared (fermented soy and sourdough, dairy from responsible farmers).

Organic products from grass-fed and happy cows should be prioritised when reintroducing dairy. Choosing dairy from goats can be a healthier option since goats are picky eaters and prefer a variety of wild grass, shrubs and leaves. If you are vegan or have sensitivities to dairy, there are fantastic coconut yoghurts available that provide a variety of probiotic strains. You can order starter cultures online and make your own yoghurt. Probiotic capsules as a supplement are an effective alternative if they are of good quality. I recommend refrigerated ones that you can buy from holistic clinicians or assorted health food shops. In my experience, the cheap ones are a waste of money and might make you believe probiotics do not work.

SUPPLEMENTATION WITH HERBS
Benefits:

- strengthens the immune system

- reduces inflammation

- increases antioxidant levels

- reduces oxidative stress

- improves lipid barrier function

Astaxanthin from algae neutralises free radicals and can counteract the inflammatory effects of the cytokine SCF [97]. Astaxanthin can be found in algae. It is the red pigment that gives salmon and shrimps their typical pink hue due to the ingestion of algae that contain astaxanthin. Algae use astaxanthin to protect themselves from UV rays as their DNA can get damaged from too much radiation exposure; it is their version of melanin. Taking an astaxanthin supplement could be beneficial to heal fibroblasts after injury from too much radiation or laser cosmetic treatments that have gone wrong.

Dr. Jules Galloway, a doctor of Naturopathic Medicine, says using zinc and an activated vitamin B complex is one of the safest ways to balance estrogen levels (zinc balances copper levels). When in doubt, she also recommends ensuring optimal liver support because low liver function compromises hormone metabolism. When this happens, your hormones get reabsorbed into your system instead of being eliminated. Remember, the liver digests fats, and your stress and sex hormones are fat-derived and therefore metabolised in your liver.

Her recommendations for liver support:

- Schisandra

- Milk thistle

- Turmeric

- B vitamins (activated)

- Dandelion root

- Liquorice root

But do not forget that no herb or supplement can fix your liver if you drink a lot of alcohol or load your system with other toxins and drugs.

If you find out through the DUTCH test that your sex hormones are out of balance, Dr. Carrie Jones, who is specialised in hormone imbalances, recommends vitex. Vitex is an adaptogen for the ovaries. It can balance progesterone and estrogen whilst being safe to use (not in pregnancy). She also recommends rhodiola, ashwagandha and American ginseng as adaptogens for the adrenals. Please get high-quality products. There are cheap ones available online, but low-quality products can contain by-products that can overburden your liver. Please dose according to the recommendations. Higher amounts do not mean better results.

SUNSHINE FOR A RADIANT BODY FROM WITHIN

SUNBATHING

Benefits:

- vitamin D production

- vitamin D has an anti-carcinogenic effect [2]

- vitamin D is anti-inflammatory [2]

- conversion of cholesterol to vitamin D3 [184]

- serotonin production

- melatonin production

- estrogen production

- improves mitochondrial function

- reduces oxidative stress

- improves hydration

The sun is an ancient healer for your body, mind, spirit and, of course, your skin. We know the benefits of vitamin D production for bone health and how happy spending time in the sunshine makes us. In Part II, "How Estrogen is Made in the Body", I have touched on how sunlight stimulates hormone production by entering light through the eyes to the brain. If we did not have sun exposure, it would deprive us of the ability to build serotonin, melatonin, dopamine and estrogen. Hormone production is triggered by the action of the visible light spectrum. The red light of the visible light spectrum also improves the function of the mitochondria, which in turn reduces oxidative stress.

Furthermore, when sunlight (mostly near infrared) hits the skin, it initiates a photochemical process in the body to make water. The energy of red light can convert liquid water (H_2O) in the body into the more viscous form of cellular water (H_3O–the fourth phase of water). The same principle is used in red light therapy for cosmetic purposes in beauty salons and medical spas to improve skin hydration.

UV light as the invisible part of the sunlight spectrum has the ability to convert cholesterol in the body to vitamin D [184], which has bone-strengthening benefits, and anti-inflammatory and anti-cancerogenic properties [2]. It takes a person with fair skin about 30 min to release 50,000 IU (1,25 mg) in the midday sun [227]. People with darker skin need a bit longer as they have fewer vitamin D receptors than fair skinned people. Again, UV light is only dangerous if used in excess. A report from the WHO (World Health Organisation) in 2006 stated that only 0.1% of the global burden of disease is attributed to excessive UV exposure. On the other hand, too little UV exposure was considered to be responsible for a much larger proportion of the global burden of disease [227]. But how much of the golden, warm rays are needed, and how much is too much?

FACTORS TO CONSIDER:

Time of the Day

Please limit sunbathing during peak hours (when the sun is at 90°/zenith) to the recommended minutes in the table below, especially if you have not built up a tan yet. Very high levels of UV emission during peak hours can potentially burn your skin. Use the morning or late afternoon hours to stay safe in the sun for longer exposures, depending on the time of the year.

Time of the Year and Location

Depending on your location and the season, there are different UV levels (defined by an index ranging from 1 to 15) during the day due to the angle of the sun shining down on the Earth's surface. I find it easiest to use the app "UV Index" to find out the current UV emission. I use the sun when the index is below five and avoid being out when the UV index is above 5. This generally means it is best to avoid unprotected sun exposure from 10 am to 4 pm during the hottest summer months (heat comes from infrared light and is not an indicator of UV levels). During the winter months, the sun is much less intense between 10 am and 12 pm and sun exposure is somewhat safer. Some experts do not recommend unprotected sun exposure above UV index 3, but UV index above 3 provides a better chance to create vitamin D. Also, UVB is considered to be more damaging than UVA and often feared, but UVB is also the range of wavelength needed to make Vitamin D. The solution to this dilemma is to adjust your exposure time to your skin's resilience.

Length of Exposure and Skin Type

It is good to know your skin type according to the Fitzpatrick scale to know how long you can stay safely in the sun. The Fitzpatrick scale is named after the dermatologist Dr. Fitzpatrick, who has contributed meaningful insights into the field of dermatology. The Fitzpatrick scale is a very helpful tool to determine skin resilience. The table below shows how long you can stay in the sun during peak hours when you are unprotected without getting sunburnt. Once you have established a tan, you can stay longer. Add a few minutes every day.

	I	II	III	IV	V	VI
HERITAGE	North European/ Irish	North European/ Swedish	Mediter- ranean	East Asian/ Indian	Indian/ South American/ African	African
EXPOSURE	5-10 mins	10-20 mins	15-25 mins	20-30 mins	30-40 mins	40-60 mins

Table 12: Safe unprotected exposure times for each skin type.

Frequency of Sun Bathing

1. Sunbathe daily to build a sun protection base (tan).

Build up gradually. The better you build up your protection during spring, the less likely you will burn in the summer. The more you maintain healthy sun exposure in summer, the more vitamin D you store to stay healthy and happy in the sun-deprived winter months.

Sun Protection

1. Avoid toxic and synthetic ingredients in your skincare routine. They can react with the sunlight and cause damage and inflammation to the skin.

2. Wide-brimmed hats and thin long linen clothes offer the best sun protection.

3. Eat foods that contain a lot of pigment, like berries, kale and even dark chocolate. They have amazing sun protection properties. In fact, they possess those colours not just to accomplish photosynthesis but also to protect themselves from sun exposure because plants and trees are immobile and cannot seek shade.

4. Choose to stay in the shade whenever possible during peak hours.

5. If you use sunscreen, I recommend zinc sunscreens without chemicals. Remember that many chemical sun filters are endocrine disruptors. Raspberry seed oil and seabuckthorn oil naturally have sun protection properties.

6. Avoid eating synthetic food additives and polyunsaturated oils (PUFAs). They can react with the sun and cause pigmentation.

I am practising this protocol and can say that in almost eight years of living in Australia, I have never had a sunburn the entire time, and I am not using sunscreen unless I am in the water for hours. If you still happen to get burned, cool the skin with a cold compress to neutralise the heat (it is the energy that is absorbed in the skin that causes the damage), apply aloe vera and seabuckthorn oil and take a high dose of vitamin C supplement to reduce the inflammation. Zinc also helps with wound healing.

App to track the UV in your region: "UV Index"

App to estimate optimum times for vitamin D production: "Dminder"

SUN GAZING

Benefits:

- improved circadian rhythm

- better melatonin production

- improved hormonal health

- increased mitochondrial health

- improved mood

- a deeper spiritual connection

The eyes are the entry point for the sunlight to travel to the brain. From there, the sunlight's electrical energy is converted to chemical energy to set off hormone production in the pineal and pituitary glands. Retina cells (cells in the eye) contain large amounts of mitochondria, which increases the ability to respond to light. This is why light therapy with red and infrared light applied to the eyes is particularly beneficial for mitochondrial health. Sun gazing is an ancient health practice that is safe when done correctly and it is for free.

There are different protocols available. As a rule of thumb, stay within one hour after sunrise and one hour before sunset to ensure safety, as no UV light is received during that window. Do not wear contact lenses or sunglasses. Stand firmly with both bare feet on the ground to allow optimum energy flow.

Here is one example of a protocol:

On the first day, gaze for 10 seconds at the sun. Then continue each day by adding 10 seconds until you reach 15 minutes of sun gazing in total. You can then reverse and subtract 10 seconds each day until you are back at 5 minutes. Then continue with 5 minutes each day of sungazing.

HEALING YOUR MITOCHONDRIA

Benefits:

- production of powerful endogenous antioxidants » reduces oxidative stress

- reduces inflammation

- improves nervous system health

- strengthens your immune system

- healing of damaged cells

9 METHODS TO INCREASE MITOCHONDRIAL HEALTH AND REDUCE OXIDATIVE STRESS:

1. Exercising

Some of your cells contain thousands of mitochondria that produce energy for the body. Most cells contain several mitochondria but red blood cells, for example, have none. A heart muscle cell contains about 5000 mitochondria, while a liver cell has around 2000. Muscle cells, including heart muscle cells, hold the most mitochondria due to their energy requirements. The more active and strong your musculature, the more active mitochondria you have, with the benefit of producing lots of endogenous antioxidants [228]. There is no need to overdo physical exercise to take advantage of that perk. Overexercising can even cause oxidative stress [229].

Short bursts of training that get your heart pumping and make you sweat, like sprints, jumps and aerobics are all great for cellular and mitochondrial health.

2. Fasting

Research shows that time restricted eating maintains mitochondrial function and endogenous antioxidant production [230][231].

3. Hot and Cold Therapy

Studies have demonstrated that heat stimulates the release of heat shock proteins that protect the mitochondria from damage [232][233]. Heat also improves the breathing capacity of mitochondria [233]. Sauna, red light therapy and exercising are gentle but effective ways to increase the body temperature without overheating. Cold stress like ice bathing or a cold shower can increase the production of new mitochondria and improve their function by increasing the production of the protein PGC-1α, a key regulator of cell metabolism [234]. Sauna and ice plunging have a long historical tradition across Europe. In ancient Rome and Greece, water therapy in thermal pools was highly regarded to heal men after battles. Sauna and bathing in hot springs or ice pools have always been a tradition among Swedes, Finns and Russians to strengthen the immune system. Whether European ancestors knew about mitochondria is unknown, but they certainly had a well established understanding and observance of the human body.

4. Sunbathing and Sungazing `

Red light in the visible and infrared spectrum has the ability to activate mitochondria [235][236]. When natural sunlight hits the body, 50% of the warming infrared light is absorbed by the mitochondria [237]. Infrared deeply penetrates through the skin to reach into the deeper tissues. Most of our mitochondria are located in our muscle, nerve, kidney, retina and liver cells. Therefore, those organs are most responsive to sunlight and should be exposed to light to activate mitochondrial function [238].

5. Avoid Blue Light

Blue light has the opposite effect on mitochondria to what red light does; it shuts the activity down. Avoid too much artificial light and screentime.

6. Eat and Drink Well

Mitochondria need nutrients for optimum function [239]. Aim for a balanced diet with:

Vitamins & Minerals:

Vit B 12: nori algae, tempeh, mushrooms [240].

Vit B 1,2,3,5,6,7,9: spinach, brown rice, lentils, oranges, avocados [241].

Vit C: peppers, citrus fruits, strawberries, broccoli [242].

Vit E: nuts, seeds, nut butters [243].

Selenium: brazil nuts, brown rice, oats, spinach, lentils [244].

Zinc: seeds, nuts, tofu, tempeh [245]. Oysters have about 60–70 times more zinc than plant foods [246].

7. Sleep Well

Mitochondria are sensitive to circadian rhythms. This is due to the adaption of human physiology to day and night times, allowing us to live in symbiosis with the environment. This adaptation is disrupted by recent changes in our lifestyles, e.g., working at night and using artificial light after sunset, which subsequently disrupts our circadian rhythm and sleep patterns. Studies on mice confirmed that chronic sleep deprivation leads to a significant decrease in mitochondrial function [247][248]. One of the most critical factors to sleeping well is melatonin. Your pineal gland releases this sleep hormone in the evening if you had sufficient sunlight in the morning and only a minimum of artificial light after sunset. It is also important to start winding down 2 hours before sleep because high cortisol levels can keep you awake.

8. Breathe Well

Insufficient oxygen supply (hypoxia) shuts down mitochondrial function. Breathe through your nose, slow and deep. Try to take five full breaths per minute. Four seconds into your nose while expanding your belly, 8 seconds out while contracting your belly.

9. Keep your Liver Clean and your Heart Happy

As mentioned before, there are thousands of mitochondria in liver and heart cells. Since the liver is a filtering organ, it is counterproductive to overburden it with toxins from food, cosmetics, smoking, alcohol and medications (that are not essential for survival).

You might wonder why we should put so much effort into our daily habits to produce those antioxidants if we can just get a supplement or an IV drip. Well, why would we choose the artificial way if we can have it for free, safely and naturally? I genuinely believe that creating balance in your body and supporting your own magnificent system is the only way to reach true and sustained health. There is nothing wrong with getting a little bit of extra support, but without the commitment to a healthy lifestyle, we cannot achieve optimum health. Furthermore, processes within the cells are highly complex and still not fully understood. Thus, there is a potential risk when intervening in these delicate systems and doing more harm than good.

COSMETICS

Cosmetic products are a beautiful addition to a daily pampering regime. Most of us love the silky textures and redolent scents of lotions, potions and creams. When choosing cosmetics for melasma, I suggest following a gentle approach. The goal is to support the healing of the skin, rather than trying to remove the hyperpigmented patches with cosmetics. Treating melasma with cosmetics alone rarely achieves the desired results, especially in the long term. Most people with melasma who have tried conventional anti-pigment products can confirm that melasma did not fade at all or at least that it came back. In saying this, there are numerous botanical ingredients that can accelerate the turnover of pigment, while your body is healing from imbalances. Melasma patients who decide to go the route of conventional medicine can have success with topically applied prescription drugs, such as hydroquinone and tretinoin. However, without a holistic healing approach, it is unlikely that the hyperpigmented areas are gone for good.

Since melasma is an inflammatory skin condition, it is important not to add more stress to the skin. Clean and organic cosmetics should be the number one choice. Reducing inflammation, as well as rebuilding the skin barrier should be the focus. The regime does not have to be elaborate. It can be a two-step or a four-step system, whatever suits your lifestyle. I recommend at least a two-step system with cleansing and moisturising at am and pm.

A two-step skincare regime if it has to be quick and easy:

1. Cleanse in the morning to remove excreted toxins from the night.

   Cleanse in the evening to remove pollution from the day to avoid oxidative stress.

2. Apply a moisturiser in the morning to protect the skin from the climate and pollution.

   Apply moisturiser in the evening to support the healing.

If you have the time or love a more elaborate daily regime, you can add a serum with active ingredients to apply underneath your moisturiser and eye cream. Encapsulated vitamin C, for example, is a great anti-pigment and antioxidant ingredient.

EXFOLIATION

While healing melasma, I do not recommend exfoliation with scrubs, or AHA like glycolic or lactic acid. The question is, does your skin need exfoliation? Most often, melasma-affected skin has its barrier function compromised, which is a contraindication towards exfoliation. If the skin feels rough or is congested, I recommend either an enzyme-based exfoliant (fruit enzyme from pineapple, for example) or a mask made of clay (bentonite clay) with a herbal infusion of arnica or calendula to take off excess skin cell buildup. Clay is cleansing and detoxifies without irritating the skin. You can add a bit of enzyme powder to the clay mask to increase the exfoliation strength. Those alternatives are super effective but much gentler, and clay has the ability to pull toxins out of tissues.

INGREDIENTS

No matter where on this planet you live, every region has wonderful herbs that help you to alleviate skin inflammation. Herbs can be used for facial steaming (not too hot) or as an infusion to mix into a clay mask. Herbs and plant extracts in products add powerful active ingredients to cleansers and moisturisers.

Here are the best anti-inflammatory ingredients:

- Aloe vera (if the climate where you live allows, grow an aloe vera plant in your home)

- Arnica

- Calendula

- Chamomile

- Liquorice root

- Pineapple enzyme (Bromelain)

- Willow bark (aspirin is made from it, avoid it if you are allergic to aspirin)

- Witch hazel

- Yarrow

- Scullcap (reduces pigmentation and lipid peroxidation [249][250])

ESSENTIAL OILS

Essential oils are Mother Earth's medicines in a bottle. They have excellent healing properties and are valuable remedies in our household and skincare. Caution should be taken when applying essential oils to the skin. Essential oils are highly concentrated plant extracts, are very potent and therefore require dilution. No more than 2% should be used in skin care applications. I primarily use 1% for the face and 2% for the body; 1ml is 20 drops of oil. Some oils are phototoxic, which may lead to an increased risk of sunburn when the skin is exposed to the sun. Phototoxic essential oils that are better used at nighttime include lavender, orange, grapefruit and bergamot.

When you mix your own cosmetics, please get some advice. There are some really good books about the safe application of essential oils.

Anti-inflammatory Essential Oils:

- German chamomile

- Roman chamomile

- Geranium

- Helichrysum

- Lavender

- Yarrow

Book recommendations: "Advanced Aromatherapy: The Science of Essential Oil Therapy" by Kurt Schnaubelt PhD.

"Essential Oil Safety: A Guide for Health Care Professionals" by Robert Tisserand & Rodney Young

PRODUCTS

Products for sensitive skin are a great choice as they have anti-inflammatory ingredients. If you want to include anti-ageing, be assured that when you reduce inflammation, you are practicing one of the best anti-ageing strategy possible. Inflammation is a major ager for your skin

If your budget does not allow you to buy products, you can use local honey to cleanse and organic coconut oil to moisturise your skin.

A few examples of clean, organic and trustworthy cosmetic brands:

Miod Organic Skincare

Mukti Organics

Living Libations

Side note:

Many cosmetic products for pigmentation contain tyrosinase inhibitors. Since modern research has identified that the overactivity of this enzyme causes hyperpigmentation, the attempt to inhibit the activity sounds logical. However, tyrosinase is just one component of a wide range of contributing factors. Inhibiting only one symptom is a Sisyphean task. It is like trying to fix water damage in the house by repetitively soaking up water instead of repairing the pipe. To follow a root cause based approach, we must identify and eliminate the factors that cause the increase of tyrosinase activity.

Book recommendations: "Renegade Beauty" by Nadine Artemis

"High Vibrational Beauty" by Kerrilynn Pamer & Cindy D Morisse

"Whole Beauty" by Shiva Rose

FREQUENCY HEALING
"Future medicine will be the medicine of frequencies." – Albert Einstein

Benefits:

- regulates the nervous system
- balances the endocrine system
- reduces inflammation
- regains body homeostasis

ANCIENT BELIEFS
Ancient Egyptians were obsessed with cosmic order and terrified of chaos. According to anecdotal evidence, Egyptians believed that chaos in the atoms is the origin of all diseases.

Each of your cells is made up of molecules; small chemical compounds that are a combination of different elements. Each of these elements is made up of spinning atoms. This creates a vibration that ripples out at a certain frequency. A frequency is defined by how often a soundwave travels through a certain point for a unit of time (frequencies are measured in Hertz). Egyptians believed that the body is in its best state when the atoms are vibrating in harmony and at the right frequency.

WE ARE BEINGS OF FREQUENCY

There are different sources and mediums from which we can receive healing frequencies, either through various forms of energy or sound. Every single object of matter that exists in our universe carries a frequency. Humans, plants, other animals, rocks, the earth, the sun, etc.

Frequency healing through energy can be delivered via various mediums, like other humans through reiki or touch therapy and massage. We all have experienced the healing and comforting energy that dogs and other pets can transfer. Dolphin Therapy is based on frequency healing. Homeopathy is based on the healing power of the vibrational energy of plants, as well as flower essences (Bachblueten) and essential oils. The plants we eat carry vibrational information.

The Earth's frequency, also called the Schumann frequency, resonates with the frequency 7.83Hz and can be felt by just being grounded on the Earth. Ever wondered why we feel so good when we are in nature? As we have evolved with the Earth's frequency, our health is directly linked to the natural frequency of our environment. Those are easily disturbed by man-made electromagnetic frequencies (EMF). The Earth's frequency of 7.83Hz is the same frequency that resonates with the sacred sound OM (the mantra of the third eye chakra) as well as the alpha and theta brainwaves. Those brainwaves promote a relaxed, dreamy mood and support cell regeneration. Theta brainwaves match the frequencies of a child's brain resonance until they are about seven years old.

Crystals carry powerful healing frequencies, and their potent effects on human well-being are widely used in alternative healing therapies. The frequency of high-quality spring water is very healing and invigorating. Have you ever heard of the holy water of Lourdes? Water can store information about prayer, songs and loving words. That is the reason why we are so susceptible to frequencies, as our bodies are made of up to 75% water by weight.

FREQUENCY HEALING WITH SOUND

Sound is received by the ears as vibrations and converted to electrical impulses. These impulses travel via the nervous system to the brain. Once the frequencies of those vibrations have reached the brain, brainwaves are altered and a cascade of effects positively or negatively impacts the bodily cells. We have all felt the invigorating or calming effects of music or chills and goosebumps. There are six ancient healing sounds that were discovered by Joseph Puleo in the 70s. With the use of a Pythagorean method, he unravelled six mathematically encoded patterns found in the Bible. Those frequencies are called Solfeggio sounds and represent the notes Do - Re - Mi - Fa - So - La - Ti. The Solfeggio sounds are found to share their fundamental character with ancient Gregorian and Indian Sanskrit chants [251]. Each of the different sounds is meant to interact with the different vibrational energies of the body as they resonate with the different chakras.

A research team in Japan evaluated the effects on the stress response by using the healing Solfeggio frequency of 528Hz on nine subjects. They found that cortisol (stress hormone) levels significantly decreased and oxytocin levels (the love hormone) increased [252]. The note of 528Hz is also called the "love frequency" or "miracle note".

A relatively new technology of frequency healing was recently realised with the development of modern devices, such as the "Healy" and "Spooky2". I have a Healy device and can absolutely recommend it. The effects on well-being are instant and profound. No wifi or Bluetooth is needed to run the programs. Such devices are more costly than playing music and certainly do not appeal to everyone. Still, they are a wonderful addition to the healing modalities and are certainly loved by tech fans.

Movie Recommendation: "Resonance – Beings of Frequency"

EARTHING

We are designed to be in nature and to physically touch the ground with our bare skin. When the free electrons of the Earth's surface are flowing through our skin into our bodies, we synchronise with the natural frequency of the Earth, and that is when we feel our best. Have you ever noticed that you feel so much better after a swim in the ocean or lake or after a walk in the bush or forest?

Earthing has plenty of benefits: reduction of pain and stress, improvement of sleep and mood, reduction of signs of osteoporosis, improved thyroid function, glucose regulation, stronger immunity and healthier looking skin [253]. In a 2014 study, earthing has shown to increase blood circulation in the face [254]. Better blood circulation means better oxygen and nutrient supply for radiant skin whilst improving skin tissue repair. Therefore, earthing can be helpful in banishing melasma, since there are plenty of clues that insufficient oxygen supply to the skin is a contributing factor to this skin condition ("Air Pollution", "The Evidence of Oxidative Stress in Melasma", "Hypoxia and Melasma").

When your cells vibrate at a harmonious frequency, your body, mind and spirit are in balance. Healing with frequency is a powerful modality for recovery and can have remarkable effects on your skin health, radiance and even the aging process. It has no side effects, is not too expensive, does not require medical supervision and promotes self-healing by simply bringing the most powerful healing tool – your body – into balance.

SUMMARY PART IV

1. Identify and test for imbalances:

• Hormones

• Heavy metals

• Gut microbiome

• Food sensitivities/gene testing

2. Detox your body and environment from environmental toxins:

• Endocrine disruptors

• Medications

• Food additives and pesticides

• Mold

• Polluted air

• Artificial light

• Heavy metals

3. Heal and nourish your body with:

• Emotional healing and stress reduction

• Organic and nutrient-dense food

• Drinking spring water, bathing and swimming in an ocean, lake or river water

• Herbs

• Sunshine

• Breathing fresh air

• Movement

- Sleep

- Natural and organic cosmetics

- Healing frequencies

- Connecting with mother earth

CONCLUSION

With the contents of this book, I hope to have evoked an inner spark in you to find strength in fighting melasma and view this skin condition in a new light. I hope it has educated you in a way that gave you a deeper understanding of your body. This book is there to empower you in taking control of your own health.

The findings of the clinical research on melasma seem to raise more questions than reaching solid and absolute conclusions. What once was identified as melasma, a pigmentary disorder caused by excess estrogen during pregnancy, has now become a skin condition that affects a broader scope of the population. Recently, melasma seems to be caused by environmental factors. Therefore, we may have to subdivide melasma into different categories, such as pregnancy melasma, environmental melasma and emotional melasma.

While we cannot narrow down one single factor that causes melasma, the evidence provided is enough to deliver a message that there is a dysregulation in the body and the dark patches are a cry for help. Therefore, re-examining and adjusting lifestyle choices to regain homeostasis is crucial in improving melasma. We also must wake up to the reality that human pollution, as well as a stressed and traumatised society, negatively affects our health, which is most likely the reason for the rise of skin disorders.

We cannot entirely avoid exposure to environmental toxins or shield ourselves from life's challenges. I am aware it can be exhausting to be vigilant about possible threats in our daily life while enjoying ourselves. But we can become more conscious of our inner and outer environment and do the best we can to improve the connection with our body, mind, spirit and planet. If we master a better connection to Mother Earth, we have a chance to contribute to her healing, which will permit us a true chance to heal our bodies.

REFERENCES

1. Sarkar R, Puri P, Jain RK, Singh A, Desai A. Melasma in men: a clinical, aetiological and histological study. J Eur Acad Dermatol Venereol. 2010;24:768–72.

2. Slominski AT, Zmijewski MA, Skobowiat C, Zbytek B, Slominski RM, Steketee JD. Sensing the environment: regulation of local and global homeostasis by the skin's neuroendocrine system. Adv Anat Embryol Cell Biol. 2012;212:v, vii, 1–115.

3. Yeung H, Kahn B, Ly BC, Tangpricha V. Dermatologic conditions in transgender populations. Endocrinol Metab Clin North Am. 2019;48:429–40.

4. Few Sunscreens Shield From UVA Rays | Environmental Working Group [Internet]. [cited 2021 Oct 7]. Available from: https://www.ewg.org/news-insights/news-release/few-sunscreens-shield-uva-rays

5. Handel AC, Miot LDB, Miot HA. Melasma: a clinical and epidemiological review. An Bras Dermatol. 2014;89:771–82.

6. Grimes PE, Yamada N, Bhawan J. Light Microscopic, Immunohistochemical, and Ultrastructural Alterations in Patients with Melasma. The American Journal of Dermatopathology. 2005;27:96–101.

7. Sanchez NP, Pathak MA, Sato S, Fitzpatrick TB, Sanchez JL, Mihm MC. Melasma: a clinical, light microscopic, ultrastructural, and immunofluorescence study. J Am Acad Dermatol. 1981;4:698–710.

8. Lee DJ, Lee J, Ha J, Park K-C, Ortonne J-P, Kang HY. Defective barrier function in melasma skin. Journal of the European Academy of Dermatology and Venereology. 2012;26:1533–7.

9. Choi JR, Won CH, Oh ES, An J, Chang SE. Does Altered Basement Membrane of Melasma Lesion Affect Treatment Outcome in Asian Skin? The American Journal of Dermatopathology. 2013;35:137–8.

10. Torres-Álvarez B, Mesa-Garza IG, Castanedo-Cázares JP, Fuentes-Ahumada C, Oros-Ovalle C, Navarrete-Solis J, et al. Histochemical and immunohistochemical study in melasma: evidence of damage in the basal membrane. Am J Dermatopathol. 2011;33:291–5.

11. Achar A, Rathi SK. Melasma: a clinico-epidemiological study of 312 cases. Indian J Dermatol. 2011;56:380–2.

12. Tamega A de A, Miot LDB, Bonfietti C, Gige TC, Marques MEA, Miot HA. Clinical patterns and epidemiological characteristics of facial melasma in Brazilian women. J Eur Acad Dermatol Venereol. 2013;27:151–6.

13. Hexsel D, Lacerda DA, Cavalcante AS, Machado Filho CAS, Kalil CLPV, Ayres EL, et al. Epidemiology of melasma in Brazilian patients: a multicenter study. Int J Dermatol. 2014;53:440–4.

14. Ortonne JP, Arellano I, Berneburg M, Cestari T, Chan H, Grimes P, et al. A global survey of the role of ultraviolet radiation and hormonal influences in the development of melasma. J Eur Acad Dermatol Venereol. 2009;23:1254–62.

15. Çakmak SK, Özcan N, Kılıç A, Koparal S, Artüz F, Çakmak A, et al. Etiopathogenetic factors, thyroid functions and thyroid autoimmunity in melasma patients. Postepy Dermatol Alergol. 2015;32:327–30.

16. Guinot C, Cheffai S, Latreille J, Dhaoui MA, Youssef S, Jaber K, et al. Aggravating factors for melasma: a prospective study in 197 Tunisian patients. J Eur Acad Dermatol Venereol. 2010;24:1060–9.

17. Romani J. Dermatology, 3rd ed. Jean L. Bolognia, Joseph L. Jorizzo, Julie V. Schaffer. 3.a ed. 2012. Editorial Saunders, Reino Unido. ISBN-13:9780723435716; 2.494 pages. Actas Dermo-Sifiliograficas (English Edition). 2012;103.

18. Mahmood K, Nadeem M, Aman S, Hameed A, Kazmi AH. Role of estrogen, progesterone and prolactin in the etiopathogenesis of melasma in females. Journal of Pakistan Association of Dermatology. 2016;21:241–7.

19. Slominski AT, Zmijewski MA, Plonka PM, Szaflarski JP, Paus R. How UV Light Touches the Brain and Endocrine System Through Skin, and Why. Endocrinology. 2018;159:1992–2007.

20. Katsarou-Katsare A, Filippou A, Theoharides TC. Effect of Stress and Other Psychological Factors on the Pathophysiology and Treatment of Dermatoses. Int J Immunopathol Pharmacol. SAGE Publications Ltd; 1999;12:205873929901200100.

21. Slominski A, Tobin DJ, Shibahara S, Wortsman J. Melanin Pigmentation in Mammalian Skin and Its Hormonal Regulation. Physiological Reviews. American Physiological Society; 2004;84:1155–228.

22. Chen Y, Lyga J. Brain-Skin Connection: Stress, Inflammation and Skin Aging. Inflamm Allergy Drug Targets. 2014;13:177–90.

23. Yaar M, Park H-Y. Melanocytes: A Window into the Nervous System. Journal of Investigative Dermatology. 2012;132:835–45.

24. Bak H, Lee HJ, Chang S-E, Choi J-H, Kim MN, Kim BJ. Increased expression of nerve growth factor receptor and neural endopeptidase in the lesional skin of melasma. Dermatol Surg. 2009;35:1244–50.

25. Purves D, Augustine GJ, Fitzpatrick D, Katz LC, LaMantia A-S, McNamara JO, et al. Trigeminal Chemoreception. Neuroscience 2nd edition [Internet]. Sinauer Associates; 2001 [cited 2020 Dec 24]; Available from: https://www.ncbi.nlm.nih.gov/books/NBK11036/

26. Calissano RL-M Pietro. The Nerve-Growth Factor: A New Tool for Manipulating Neurons [Internet]. Scientific American. [cited 2022 Mar 28]. Available from: https://www.scientificamerican.com/article/the-nerve-growth-factor/

27. Aloe L, Skaper SD, Leon A, Levi-Montalcini R. Nerve Growth Factor and Autoimmune Diseases. Autoimmunity. Taylor & Francis; 1994;19:141–50.

28. Levi-Montalcini R, Skaper SD, Toso RD, Petrelli L, Leon A. Nerve growth factor: from neurotrophin to neurokine. Trends in Neurosciences. Elsevier; 1996;19:514–20.

29. Bonini S, Lambiase A, Bonini S, Angelucci F, Magrini L, Manni L, et al. Circulating nerve growth factor levels are increased in humans with allergic diseases and asthma. Proc Natl Acad Sci U S A. 1996;93:10955–60.

30. Bonini S, Lambiase A, Bonini S, Levi-Schaffer F, Aloe L. Nerve growth factor: an important molecule in allergic inflammation and tissue remodelling. Int Arch Allergy Immunol. 1999;118:159–62.

31. Yaar M, Grossman K, Eller M, Gilchrest BA. Evidence for nerve growth factor-mediated paracrine effects in human epidermis. J Cell Biol. 1991;115:821–8.

32. Scholzen T, Armstrong CA, Bunnett NW, Luger TA, Olerud JE, Ansel JC. Neuropeptides in the skin: interactions between the neuroendocrine and the skin immune systems. Exp Dermatol. 1998;7:81–96.

33.   Byun JW, Park IS, Choi GS, Shin J. Role of fibroblast-derived factors in the pathogenesis of melasma. Clin Exp Dermatol. 2016;41:601–9.

34.   Chen Z, Chen F, Fang Z, Zhao H, Zhan C, Li C, et al. Glial activation and inflammation in the NTS in a rat model after exposure to diesel exhaust particles. Environ Toxicol Pharmacol. 2021;83:103584.

35.   Barker JS, Wu Z, Hunter DD, Dey RD. Ozone Exposure Initiates a Sequential Signaling Cascade in Airways Involving Interleukin-1beta Release, Nerve Growth Factor Secretion, and Substance P Upregulation. J Toxicol Environ Health A. 2015;78:397–407.

36.   Alleva E, Aloe L, Bigi S. An updated role for nerve growth factor in neurobehavioural regulation of adult vertebrates. Rev Neurosci. 1993;4:41–62.

37.   Alleva E, Santucci D. Psychosocial vs. "physical" stress situations in rodents and humans: role of neurotrophins. Physiol Behav. 2001;73:313–20.

38.   Aloe L, Bracci-Laudiero L, Alleva E, Lambiase A, Micera A, Tirassa P. Emotional stress induced by parachute jumping enhances blood nerve growth factor levels and the distribution of nerve growth factor receptors in lymphocytes. Proc Natl Acad Sci U S A. 1994;91:10440–4.

39.   Alleva E, Aloe L, Cirulli F, Della Seta D, Tirassa P. Serum NGF levels increase during lactation and following maternal aggression in mice. Physiol Behav. 1996;59:461–6.

40.   Rizzo AM, Berselli P, Zava S, Montorfano G, Negroni M, Corsetto P, et al. Endogenous antioxidants and radical scavengers. Adv Exp Med Biol. 2010;698:52–67.

41.   Clarke G, Grenham S, Scully P, Fitzgerald P, Moloney RD, Shanahan F, et al. The microbiome-gut-brain axis during early life regulates the hippocampal serotonergic system in a sex-dependent manner. Mol Psychiatry. 2013;18:666–73.

42.   Neuman H, Debelius JW, Knight R, Koren O. Microbial endocrinology: the interplay between the microbiota and the endocrine system. FEMS Microbiol Rev. 2015;39:509–21.

43.   de Bold AJ, Borenstein HB, Veress AT, Sonnenberg H. A rapid and potent natriuretic response to intravenous injection of atrial myocardial extract in rats. Life Sci. 1981;28:89–94.

44.   Nakagawa Y, Nishikimi T, Kuwahara K. Atrial and brain natriuretic peptides: Hormones secreted from the heart. Peptides. 2019;111:18–25.

45.   Endocrine System: Illustrations of Anatomy, Function, Organs & Glands [Internet]. eMedicineHealth. [cited 2020 May 28]. Available from: https://www.emedicinehealth.com/anatomy_of_the_endocrine_system/article_em.htm

46.   Thyroid Autoantibodies (TPOAb, TgAb and TRAb) [Internet]. Medscape. [cited 2020 Jun 8]. Available from: http://www.medscape.com/viewarticle/452668

47.   Slominski A, Baker J, Ermak G, Chakraborty A, Pawelek J. Ultraviolet B stimulates production of corticotropin releasing factor (CRF) by human melanocytes. FEBS Lett. 1996;399:175–6.

48.   Slominski A, Zbytek B, Szczesniewski A, Semak I, Kaminski J, Sweatman T, et al. CRH stimulation of corticosteroids production in melanocytes is mediated by ACTH. Am J Physiol Endocrinol Metab. 2005;288:E701-706.

49.   Wolf R, Wolf D, Tamir A, Politi Y. Metasma: a mask of stress. British Journal of Dermatology. 1991;125:192–192.

50.   Cao J, Papadopoulou N, Kempuraj D, Boucher WS, Sugimoto K, Cetrulo CL, et al. Human mast cells express corticotropin-releasing hormone (CRH) receptors and CRH leads to selective secretion of vascular endothelial growth factor. J Immunol. 2005;174:7665–75.

51.   Slominski AT, Zmijewski MA, Zbytek B, Tobin DJ, Theoharides TC, Rivier J. Key role of CRF

in the skin stress response system. Endocr Rev. 2013;34:827–84.

52. Slominski A, Wortsman J. Neuroendocrinology of the Skin1. Endocrine Reviews. 2000;21:457–87.

53. Donald Trump Age, Height, Wife, Children, Family, Biography & More » StarsUnfolded [Internet]. [cited 2021 Oct 19]. Available from: https://starsunfolded.com/donald-trump/

54. Trump delivers a pathetic stream of lies from White House as he desperately tries to claim victory | Salon.com [Internet]. [cited 2021 Oct 19]. Available from: https://www.salon.com/2020/11/06/trump-delivers-a-pathetic-stream-of-lies-from-white-house-as-he-desperately-tries-to-claim-victory_partner/

55. Who was John F. Kennedy? Everything You Need to Know [Internet]. [cited 2021 Oct 19]. Available from: https://www.thefamouspeople.com/profiles/john-f-kennedy-50.php

56. Prince J. Glimpse into Jackie Kennedy's Life after JFK's Death: "She Was Miserable" [Internet]. news.amomama.com. 2020 [cited 2021 Oct 19]. Available from: https://news.amomama.com/228153-jackie-kennedy-was-reportedly-miserable.html

57. Maeda K, Naganuma M, Fukuda M, Matsunaga J, Tomita Y. Effect of pituitary and ovarian hormones on human melanocytes in vitro. Pigment Cell Res. 1996;9:204–12.

58. Suzuki I, Cone RD, Im S, Nordlund J, Abdel-Malek ZA. Binding of melanotropic hormones to the melanocortin receptor MC1R on human melanocytes stimulates proliferation and melanogenesis. Endocrinology. 1996;137:1627–33.

59. Dissanayake NS, Mason RS. Modulation of skin cell functions by transforming growth factor-beta1 and ACTH after ultraviolet irradiation. J Endocrinol. 1998;159:153–63.

60. Gillbro JM, Marles LK, Hibberts NA, Schallreuter KU. Autocrine catecholamine biosynthesis and the beta-adrenoceptor signal promote pigmentation in human epidermal melanocytes. J Invest Dermatol. 2004;123:346–53.

61. Song X, Shen Y, Zhou Y, Lou Q, Han L, Ho JK, et al. General hyperpigmentation induced by Grave's disease. Medicine (Baltimore) [Internet]. 2018 [cited 2021 Mar 27];97. Available from: https://www.ncbi.nlm.nih.gov/pmc/articles/PMC6310574/

62. Elbenaye J, Ouleghzal H, Elhaouri M. Periorbital hyperpigmentation in Graves disease's hyperthyroidism or "Jellinek sign." Med Clin Arch [Internet]. 2018 [cited 2021 Mar 27];2. Available from: https://www.oatext.com/periorbital-hyperpigmentation-in-graves-diseases-hyperthyroidism-or-jellinek-sign.php

63. Martin NM, Smith KL, Bloom SR, Small CJ. Interactions between the melanocortin system and the hypothalamo-pituitary-thyroid axis. Peptides. 2006;27:333–9.

64. Suzuki I, Tada A, Ollmann MM, Barsh GS, Im S, Lynn Lamoreux M, et al. Agouti Signaling Protein Inhibits Melanogenesis and the Response of Human Melanocytes to α-Melanotropin. Journal of Investigative Dermatology. 1997;108:838–42.

65. Lechan RM, Fekete C. Role of melanocortin signaling in the regulation of the hypothalamic–pituitary–thyroid (HPT) axis. Peptides. 2006;27:310–25.

66. Administration AGD of HTG. Beware the Barbie drug: the dangers of using melanotan [Internet]. Therapeutic Goods Administration (TGA). Australian Government Department of Health; 2019 [cited 2021 May 7]. Available from: https://www.tga.gov.au/behind-news/beware-barbie-drug-dangers-using-melanotan

67. Fekete C, Légrádi G, Mihály E, Huang QH, Tatro JB, Rand WM, et al. alpha-Melanocyte-stimulating hormone is contained in nerve terminals innervating thyrotropin-releasing hormone-synthesizing neurons in the hypothalamic paraventricular nucleus and prevents fasting-induced suppression of prothyrotropin-releasing hormone gene expression. J Neurosci. 2000;20:1550–8.

68. Kim MS, Small CJ, Stanley SA, Morgan DG, Seal LJ, Kong WM, et al. The central melanocortin system affects the hypothalamo-pituitary thyroid axis and may mediate the effect of leptin. J Clin Invest.

2000;105:1005–11.

69. Lutfi RJ, Fridmanis M, Misiunas AL, Pafume O, Gonzalez EA, Villemur JA, et al. Association of melasma with thyroid autoimmunity and other thyroidal abnormalities and their relationship to the origin of the melasma. J Clin Endocrinol Metab. 1985;61:28–31.

70. Rostami Mogaddam M, Iranparvar Alamdari M, Maleki N, Safavi Ardabili N, Abedkouhi S. Evaluation of autoimmune thyroid disease in melasma. J Cosmet Dermatol. 2015;14:167–71.

71. Ameneh Y, Banafsheh H. Association of Melasma with Thyroid Autoimmunity: A Case-Control Study. Iranian Journal of Dermatology. Iranian Society of Dermatology; 2010;13:51–3.

72. The Relations Between Stress, Trauma, and Autoimmune Conditions [Internet]. Well.Org. 2019 [cited 2022 Apr 1]. Available from: https://well.org/medicine/ stress-trauma-autoimmune-conditions/

73. Rozing MP, Westendorp RGJ, Maier AB, Wijsman CA, Frölich M, de Craen AJM, et al. Serum triiodothyronine levels and inflammatory cytokine production capacity. AGE. 2012;34:195–201.

74. Siddiqi A, Monson JP, Wood DF, Besser GM, Burrin JM. Serum cytokines in thyrotoxicosis. J Clin Endocrinol Metab. 1999;84:435–9.

75. Jian D, Jiang D, Su J, Chen W, Hu X, Kuang Y, et al. Diethylstilbestrol enhances melanogenesis via cAMP-PKA-mediating up-regulation of tyrosinase and MITF in mouse B16 melanoma cells. Steroids. 2011;76:1297–304.

76. Siiteri PK. Adipose tissue as a source of hormones. Am J Clin Nutr. 1987;45:277–82.

77. Hetemäki N, Mikkola TS, Tikkanen MJ, Wang F, Hämäläinen E, Turpeinen U, et al. Adipose tissue estrogen production and metabolism in premenopausal women. J Steroid Biochem Mol Biol. 2021;209:105849.

78. Romm A. The Estrobolome: The Fascinating Way Your Gut Impacts Your Estrogen Levels [Internet]. Aviva Romm, MD. 2021 [cited 2022 Sep 10]. Available from: https://avivaromm. com/estrobolome/

79. Lieberman R, Moy L. Estrogen receptor expression in melasma: results from facial skin of affected patients. J Drugs Dermatol. 2008;7:463–5.

80. Jang YH, Lee JY, Kang HY, Lee E-S, Kim YC. Oestrogen and progesterone receptor expression in melasma: an immunohistochemical analysis. J Eur Acad Dermatol Venereol. 2010;24:1312–6.

81. Jang YH, Sim JH, Kang HY, Kim YC, Lee E-S. The histopathological characteristics of male melasma: comparison with female melasma and lentigo. J Am Acad Dermatol. 2012;66:642–9.

82. Matamá T, Araújo R, Preto A, Cavaco-Paulo A, Gomes AC. In vitro induction of melanin synthesis and extrusion by tamoxifen. Int J Cosmet Sci. 2013;35:368–74.

83. Polin SA, Ascher SM. The effect of tamoxifen on the genital tract. Cancer Imaging. 2008;8:135–45.

84. Mourits MJ, De Vries EG, Willemse PH, Ten Hoor KA, Hollema H, Van der Zee AG. Tamoxifen treatment and gynecologic side effects: a review. Obstet Gynecol. 2001;97:855–66.

85. Lum SS, Woltering EA, Fletcher WS, Pommier RF. Changes in serum estrogen levels in women during tamoxifen therapy. Am J Surg. 1997;173:399–402.

86. Kim S-W, Yoon H-S. Tamoxifen-induced melasma in a postmenopausal woman. J Eur Acad Dermatol Venereol. 2009;23:1199–200.

87. Balita-crisostomo C, Frez M. Tamoxifen-induced melasma in a vitiligo patient. :1.

88. Adalatkhah H, Sadeghi Bazargani H. The Association Between Melasma and Postinflammatory Hyperpigmentation in Acne Patients. Iran Red Crescent Med J. 2013;15:400–3.

89. Hachiya A, Kobayashi A, Ohuchi A, Takema Y, Imokawa G. The Paracrine Role of Stem Cell Factor/c-kit Signaling in the Activation of Human Melanocytes in Ultraviolet-B-Induced Pigmentation.

Journal of Investigative Dermatology. 2001;116:578–86.

90. Wang Y, Viennet C, Robin S, Berthon J-Y, He L, Humbert P. Precise role of dermal fibroblasts on melanocyte pigmentation. Journal of Dermatological Science. 2017;88:159–66.

91. Imokawa G. Autocrine and paracrine regulation of melanocytes in human skin and in pigmentary disorders. Pigment Cell Res. 2004;17:96–110.

92. Kang HY, Hwang JS, Lee JY, Ahn JH, Kim J-Y, Lee E-S, et al. The dermal stem cell factor and c-kit are overexpressed in melasma. Br J Dermatol. 2006;154:1094–9.

93. Lim X, Nusse R. Wnt Signaling in Skin Development, Homeostasis, and Disease. Cold Spring Harb Perspect Biol [Internet]. 2013 [cited 2020 May 29];5. Available from: https://www.ncbi.nlm.nih.gov/pmc/articles/PMC3552514/

94. Yamamoto T, Yokozeki H. Persistent bilateral hyperpigmentation caused by local stem cell factor injection. J Eur Acad Dermatol Venereol. 2007;21:576–7.

95. Bellet JS, Obadiah JM, Frothingham BM, Kurtzberg J, Grichnik JM. A patient with extensive stem cell factor-induced hyperpigmentation. Cutis. 2003;71:149–52.

96. Grichnik JM, Burch JA, Burchette J, Shea CR. The SCF/KIT pathway plays a critical role in the control of normal human melanocyte homeostasis. J Invest Dermatol. 1998;111:233–8.

97. Niwano T, Terazawa S, Nakajima H, Imokawa G. The stem cell factor-stimulated melanogenesis in human melanocytes can be abrogated by interrupting the phosphorylation of MSK1: evidence for involvement of the p38/MSK1/CREB/MITF axis. Arch Dermatol Res. 2018;310:187–96.

98. Hernández-Barrera R, Torres-Alvarez B, Castanedo-Cazares JP, Oros-Ovalle C, Moncada B. Solar elastosis and presence of mast cells as key features in the pathogenesis of melasma. Clin Exp Dermatol. 2008;33:305–8.

99. Tomita Y, Maeda K, Tagami H. Melanocyte-stimulating properties of arachidonic acid metabolites: possible role in postinflammatory pigmentation. Pigment Cell Res. 1992;5:357–61.

100. Tomita Y, Maeda K, Tagami H. Leukotrienes and thromboxane B2 stimulate normal human melanocytes in vitro: possible inducers of postinflammatory pigmentation. Tohoku J Exp Med. 1988;156:303–4.

101. Rodríguez-Arámbula A, Torres-Álvarez B, Cortés-García D, Fuentes-Ahumada C, Castanedo-Cázares JP. CD4, IL-17, and COX-2 Are Associated With Subclinical Inflammation in Malar Melasma. The American Journal of Dermatopathology. 2015;37:761–6.

102. Essential Fatty Acids and Skin Health [Internet]. Linus Pauling Institute. 2016 [cited 2020 May 24]. Available from: https://lpi.oregonstate.edu/mic/health-disease/skin-health/essential-fatty-acids

103. Yoshida M, Takahashi Y, Inoue S. Histamine induces melanogenesis and morphologic changes by protein kinase A activation via H2 receptors in human normal melanocytes. J Invest Dermatol. 2000;114:334–42.

104. Tomita Y, Maeda K, Tagami H. Histamine stimulates normal human melanocytes in vitro: one of the possible inducers of hyperpigmentation in urticaria pigmentosa. J Dermatol Sci. 1993;6:146–54.

105. Aguilar TAF, HernándezNavarro BC, Pérez JAM. Endogenous Antioxidants: A Review of their Role in Oxidative Stress [Internet]. A Master Regulator of Oxidative Stress - The Transcription Factor Nrf2. IntechOpen; 2016 [cited 2021 Jun 11]. Available from: https://www.intechopen.com/books/a-master-regulator-of-oxidative-stress-the-transcription-factor-nrf2endogenous-antioxidants-a-review-of-their-role-in-oxidative-stress

106. Wood JM, Jimbow K, Boissy RE, Slominski A, Plonka PM, Slawinski J, et al. What's the use of generating melanin? Exp Dermatol. 1999;8:153–64.

107. Seçkin HY, Kalkan G, Baş Y, Akbaş A, Önder Y, Özyurt H, et al. Oxidative stress status in patients with melasma. Cutan Ocul Toxicol. 2014;33:212–7.

108. Sarkar R, Devadasan S, Choubey V, Goswami B. Melatonin and oxidative stress in melasma - an unexplored territory; a prospective study. Int J Dermatol. 2020;59:572–5.

109. Jo H-Y, Kim C-K, Suh I-B, Ryu S-W, Ha K-S, Kwon Y-G, et al. Co-localization of inducible nitric oxide synthase and phosphorylated Akt in the lesional skins of patients with melasma. J Dermatol. 2009;36:10–6.

110. Sasaki M, Horikoshi T, Uchiwa H, Miyachi Y. Up-regulation of Tyrosinase Gene by Nitric Oxide in Human Melanocytes. Pigment Cell Research. 2000;13:248–52.

111. Roméro-Graillet C, Aberdam E, Clément M, Ortonne JP, Ballotti R. Nitric oxide produced by ultraviolet-irradiated keratinocytes stimulates melanogenesis. J Clin Invest. 1997;99:635–42.

112. Trauma and the Pituitary [Internet]. Pituitary World News. 2017 [cited 2022 Apr 2]. Available from: https://pituitaryworldnews.org/trauma-and-the-pituitary/

113. It's Time to Talk About Trauma [Internet]. Pituitary World News. 2021 [cited 2022 Apr 2]. Available from: https://pituitaryworldnews.org/its-time-to-talk-about-trauma/

114. Dube SR, Fairweather D, Pearson WS, Felitti VJ, Anda RF, Croft JB. Cumulative Childhood Stress and Autoimmune Diseases in Adults. Psychosom Med. 2009;71:243–50.

115. Pizzino G, Irrera N, Cucinotta M, Pallio G, Mannino F, Arcoraci V, et al. Oxidative Stress: Harms and Benefits for Human Health. Oxid Med Cell Longev. 2017;2017:8416763.

116. Gender and Stress [Internet]. https://www.apa.org. [cited 2021 Oct 13]. Available from: https://www.apa.org/news/press/releases/stress/2010/gender-stress

117. Wahbeh H, Oken BS. Salivary Cortisol Lower in Posttraumatic Stress Disorder. J Trauma Stress. 2013;26:10.1002/jts.21798.

118. Writer MA-SHS. Violence and trauma in childhood accelerate puberty [Internet]. Harvard Gazette. 2020 [cited 2022 Apr 2]. Available from: https://news.harvard.edu/gazette/story/2020/08/violence-and-trauma-in-childhood-accelerate-puberty/

119. Noll JG, Trickett PK, Long JD, Negriff S, Susman EJ, Shalev I, et al. Childhood Sexual Abuse and Early Timing of Puberty. J Adolesc Health. 2017;60:65–71.

120. Peinado FM, Iribarne-Durán LM, Ocón-Hernández O, Olea N, Artacho-Cordón F. Endocrine Disrupting Chemicals in Cosmetics and Personal Care Products and Risk of Endometriosis [Internet]. Endometriosis. IntechOpen; 2020 [cited 2021 Jun 9]. Available from: https://www.intechopen.com/books/endometriosisendocrine-disrupting-chemicals-in-cosmetics-and-personal-care-products-and-risk-of-endometriosis

121. Watkins DJ, Ferguson KK, Anzalota Del Toro LV, Alshawabkeh AN, Cordero JF, Meeker JD. Associations between urinary phenol and paraben concentrations and markers of oxidative stress and inflammation among pregnant women in Puerto Rico. Int J Hyg Environ Health. 2015;218:212–9.

122. Thompson PA, Khatami M, Baglole CJ, Sun J, Harris SA, Moon E-Y, et al. Environmental immune disruptors, inflammation and cancer risk. Carcinogenesis. 2015;36 Suppl 1:S232-253.

123. ch1.pdf [Internet]. [cited 2021 Jun 11]. Available from: https://www.who.int/ipcs/publications/en/ch1.pdf

124. La Merrill MA, Vandenberg LN, Smith MT, Goodson W, Browne P, Patisaul HB, et al. Consensus on the key characteristics of endocrine-disrupting chemicals as a basis for hazard identification. Nat Rev Endocrinol. 2020;16:45–57.

125.   Dirty Dozen Endocrine Disruptors [Internet]. EWG. [cited 2020 Jun 9]. Available from: https://www.ewg.org/research/dirty-dozen-list-endocrine-disruptors

126.   EDCs Infographics 22.2.20192 Low Doses Matter.pdf [Internet]. [cited 2021 Nov 5]. Available from: http://endocrinedisruption.org/assets/media/documents/EDCs%20Infographics%20 22.2.20192%20Low%20Doses%20Matter.pdf

127.   Nailed | Environmental Working Group [Internet]. [cited 2021 Nov 5]. Available from: https://www.ewg.org/research/nailed

128.   Conti P, Tettamanti L, Mastrangelo F, Ronconi G, Frydas I, Kritas SK, et al. Impact of Fungi on Immune Responses. Clinical Therapeutics. Elsevier; 2018;40:885–8.

129.   Kritas SK, Gallenga CE, D Ovidio C, Ronconi G, Caraffa A, Toniato E, et al. Impact of mold on mast cell-cytokine immune response. J Biol Regul Homeost Agents. 2018;32:763–8.

130.   Edmondson DA, Barrios CS, Brasel TL, Straus DC, Kurup VP, Fink JN. Immune Response among Patients Exposed to Molds. Int J Mol Sci. 2009;10:5471–84.

131.   Household Mold Linked To Depression [Internet]. ScienceDaily. [cited 2022 Apr 12]. Available from: https://www.sciencedaily.com/releases/2007/08/070829162815.htm

132.   Darbre PD. Chapter 1 - What Are Endocrine Disrupters and Where Are They Found? In: Darbre PD, editor. Endocrine Disruption and Human Health [Internet]. Boston: Academic Press; 2015 [cited 2022 Apr 12]. p. 3–26. Available from: https://www.sciencedirect.com/science/article/pii/B9780128011393000016

133.   Smith M, McGinnis MR. CHAPTER 32 - Mycotoxins and their effects on humans. In: Anaissie EJ, McGinnis MR, Pfaller MA, editors. Clinical Mycology (Second Edition) [Internet]. Edinburgh: Churchill Livingstone; 2009 [cited 2022 Apr 12]. p. 649–56. Available from: https://www.sciencedirect.com/science/article/pii/B9781416056805000323

134.   Zhang G-L, Feng Y-L, Song J-L, Zhou X-S. Zearalenone: A Mycotoxin With Different Toxic Effect in Domestic and Laboratory Animals' Granulosa Cells. Front Genet. 2018;9:667.

135.   Basler RSW. Minocycline-Related Hyperpigmentation. Arch Dermatol. 1985;121:606.

136.   Mouton RW, Jordaan HF, Schneider JW. A new type of minocycline-induced cutaneous hyperpigmentation. Clin Exp Dermatol. 2004;29:8–14.

137.   Larsson BS. Interaction Between Chemicals and Melanin. Pigment Cell Research. 1993;6:127–33.

138.   Mårs U, Larsson BS. Pheomelanin as a binding site for drugs and chemicals. Pigment Cell Res. 1999;12:266–74.

139.   Greiner AC, Nicolson GA, Baker RA. Therapy of Chlorpromazine Melanosis: A Preliminary Report. Can Med Assoc J. 1964;91:636–8.

140.   Ban TA, Lehmann HE. Skin Pigmentation, A Rare Side Effect of Chlorpromazine. Canadian Psychiatric Association Journal. 1965;10:112–24.

141.   Maeda K, Tomita Y. Mechanism of the Inhibitory Effect of Tranexamic Acid on Melanogenesis in Cultured Human Melanocytes in the Presence of Keratinocyte-conditioned Medium. Journal of Health Science. 2007;53:389–96.

142.   Na JI, Choi SY, Yang SH, Choi HR, Kang HY, Park K-C. Effect of tranexamic acid on melasma: a clinical trial with histological evaluation. J Eur Acad Dermatol Venereol. 2013;27:1035–9.

143.   Jee S-H, Kuo H-W, Su WPD, Chang C-H, Sun C-C, Wang J-D. PHOTODAMAGE AND SKIN CANCER AMONG PARAQUAT WORKERS. Int J Dermatol. 1995;34:466–9.

144.   Banned In 32 Countries, Paraquat Use Is Expected To Increase In The United States. Spirit of Change Magazine | Holistic New England [Internet]. [cited 2022 Apr 15]. Available from: https://

www.spiritofchange.orgbanned-in-32-countries-paraquat-use-is-expected-to-increase-in-the-united-states/

145. Paraquat in India: too big a risk for farmers and workers | IPEN [Internet]. [cited 2022 Apr 15]. Available from: https://ipen.org/news/paraquat-india-too-big-risk-farmers-and-workers

146. Authority AP and VM. Paraquat chemical review [Internet]. Australian Pesticides and Veterinary Medicines Authority. Australian Pesticides and Veterinary Medicines Authority; 2014 [cited 2022 Apr 15]. Available from: https://apvma.gov.au/node/12666

147. Bowe W, Patel NB, Logan AC. Acne vulgaris, probiotics and the gut-brain-skin axis: from anecdote to translational medicine. Benef Microbes. 2014;5:185–99.

148. Poon VKM, Huang L, Burd A. Biostimulation of dermal fibroblast by sublethal Q-switched Nd:YAG 532 nm laser: collagen remodeling and pigmentation. J Photochem Photobiol B, Biol. 2005;81:1–8.

149. Kimura A, Kanazawa N, Li H-J, Yonei N, Yamamoto Y, Furukawa F. Influence of chemical peeling on the skin stress response system. Exp Dermatol. 2012;21 Suppl 1:8–10.

150. Roberts WE. Pollution as a risk factor for the development of melasma and other skin disorders of facial hyperpigmentation - is there a case to be made? J Drugs Dermatol. 2015;14:337–41.

151. Block ML, Calderón-Garcidueñas L. Air Pollution: Mechanisms of Neuroinflammation & CNS Disease. Trends Neurosci. 2009;32:506–16.

152. Block ML, Calderón-Garcidueñas L. Air Pollution: Mechanisms of Neuroinflammation & CNS Disease. Trends Neurosci. 2009;32:506–16.

153. Craig L, Brook JR, Chiotti Q, Croes B, Gower S, Hedley A, et al. Air Pollution and Public Health: A Guidance Document for Risk Managers. Journal of Toxicology and Environmental Health, Part A. Taylor & Francis; 2008;71:588–698.

154. Tseng C-Y, Wang J-S, Chao M-W. Causation by Diesel Exhaust Particles of Endothelial Dysfunctions in Cytotoxicity, Pro-inflammation, Permeability, and Apoptosis Induced by ROS Generation. Cardiovasc Toxicol. 2017;17:384–92.

155. Kim EH, Kim YC, Lee E-S, Kang HY. The vascular characteristics of melasma. J Dermatol Sci. 2007;46:111–6.

156. Rey S, Semenza GL. Hypoxia-inducible factor-1-dependent mechanisms of vascularization and vascular remodelling. Cardiovasc Res. 2010;86:236–42.

157. Prabhakar NR, Semenza GL. Oxygen Sensing and Homeostasis. Physiology (Bethesda). 2015;30:340–8.

158. Gao J, Ding X, Zhang Y, Dai D, Liu M, Zhang C, et al. Hypoxia/oxidative stress alters the pharmacokinetics of CPU86017-RS through mitochondrial dysfunction and NADPH oxidase activation. Acta Pharmacol Sin. Nature Publishing Group; 2013;34:1575–84.

159. Bedogni B, Powell MB. Skin Hypoxia: A Promoting Environmental Factor in Melanomagenesis. Cell Cycle. 2006;5:1258–61.

160. Hypoxemia (low blood oxygen) Causes [Internet]. Mayo Clinic. [cited 2021 Aug 9]. Available from: https://www.mayoclinic.org/symptoms/hypoxemia/basics/definition/sym-20050930

161. US Department of Commerce NO and AA. Responding to Hurricanes [Internet]. [cited 2021 Aug 9]. Available from: https://oceanservice.noaa.gov/hazards/hypoxia/

162. Liberman J. Light: Medicine of the Future: How We Can Use It to Heal Ourselves NOW. Inner Traditions / Bear & Co; 1990.

163. Bonmati-Carrion MA, Arguelles-Prieto R, Martinez-Madrid MJ, Reiter R, Hardeland R, Rol MA, et al. Protecting the Melatonin Rhythm through Circadian Healthy Light Exposure. Int J Mol Sci. 2014;15:23448–500.

164. Duffy JF, Czeisler CA. Effect of Light on Human Circadian Physiology. Sleep Med Clin.

2009;4:165-77.

165. Cos S, Martínez-Campa C, Mediavilla MD, Sánchez-Barceló EJ. Melatonin modulates aromatase activity in MCF-7 human breast cancer cells. Journal of Pineal Research. 2005;38:136-42.

166. Kong X, Gao R, Wang Z, Wang X, Fang Y, Gao J, et al. Melatonin: A Potential Therapeutic Option for Breast Cancer. Trends Endocrinol Metab. 2020;31:859-71.

167. Viswanathan AN, Hankinson SE, Schernhammer ES. Night shift work and the risk of endometrial cancer. Cancer Res. 2007;67:10618-22.

168. Mahmoud BH, Ruvolo E, Hexsel CL, Liu Y, Owen MR, Kollias N, et al. Impact of long-wavelength UVA and visible light on melanocompetent skin. J Invest Dermatol. 2010;130:2092-7.

169. Kollias N, Baqer A. An Experimental Study of the Changes in Pigmentation in Human Skin In Vivo with Visible and Near Infrared Light. undefined [Internet]. 1984 [cited 2022 Apr 24]; Available from: https://www.semanticscholar.org/paper/Visible-Light-Induces-Melanogenesis-in-Human-Skin-a-Randhawa-Seo/ce5c61b4d68191d3fa2e6df5a6b652fbe5712aba

170. Porges SB, Kaidbey KH, Grove GL. Quantification of visible light-induced melanogenesis in human skin. Photodermatol. 1988;5:197-200.

171. Duteil L, Cardot-Leccia N, Queille-Roussel C, Maubert Y, Harmelin Y, Boukari F, et al. Differences in visible light-induced pigmentation according to wavelengths: a clinical and histological study in comparison with UVB exposure. Pigment Cell Melanoma Res. 2014;27:822-6.

172. Haywood R. Relevance of sunscreen application method, visible light and sunlight intensity to free-radical protection: A study of ex vivo human skin. Photochem Photobiol. 2006;82:1123-31.

173. Liebel F, Kaur S, Ruvolo E, Kollias N, Southall MD. Irradiation of skin with visible light induces reactive oxygen species and matrix-degrading enzymes. Journal of Investigative Dermatology. 2012;132:1901-7.

174. Skobowiat C, Dowdy JC, Sayre RM, Tuckey RC, Slominski A. Cutaneous hypothalamic-pituitary-adrenal axis homolog: regulation by ultraviolet radiation. Am J Physiol Endocrinol Metab. 2011;301:E484-493.

175. Ultraviolet Radiation [Internet]. [cited 2021 Oct 7]. Available from: https://ehs.lbl.gov/resource/documents/radiation-protection/non-ionizing-radiation/ultraviolet-radiation/

176. Health C for D and R. Ultraviolet (UV) Radiation. FDA [Internet]. FDA; 2020 [cited 2021 Oct 6]; Available from: https://www.fda.gov/radiation-emitting-products/tanning?ultraviolet-uv-radiation

177. Mironava T, Hadjiargyrou M, Simon M, Rafailovich MH. The Effects of UV Emission from Compact Fluorescent Light Exposure on Human Dermal Fibroblasts and Keratinocytes In Vitro. Photochemistry and Photobiology. 2012;88:1497-506.

178. Study Reveals Harmful Effects of CFL Bulbs to Skin | | SBU News [Internet]. [cited 2022 Oct 10]. Available from: https://news.stonybrook.edu/researchstudy-reveals-harmful-effects-of-cfl-bulbs-to-skin-2/

179. Do LED Lights Emit UV Rays and Radiation? [Internet]. LampHQ [cited 2022 Oct 10]. Available from: https://lamphq.com/led-radiation/

180. Health C for D and R. Mercury Vapor Lamps (Mercury Vapor Light Bulbs). FDA [Internet]. FDA; 2020 [cited 2022 Jun 2]; Available from: https://www.fda.gov/radiation-emitting-products/home-business-and-entertainment-products/mercury-vapor-lamps-mercury-vapor-light-bulbs

181. Tuchinda C, Srivannaboon S, Lim HW. Photoprotection by window glass, automobile glass, and sunglasses. undefined [Internet]. 2006 [cited 2022 Apr 24]; Available from: https://www.semanticscholar.org/paper/Assessment-of-Levels-of-Ultraviolet-A-Light-in-and-Wachler/5c8211bf1e64bf92c3784bec5d893d04f7705e30

182. Aljaff PM, Rasheed BO, Muhammad KK. Evaluation of Solar Radiation Transmission through

Window glasses and Transparent Facades for Buildings in Sulaimani. 2018.

183. Boxer Wachler BS. Assessment of Levels of Ultraviolet A Light Protection in Automobile Windshields and Side Windows. JAMA Ophthalmol. 2016;134:772–5.

184. Chaitanya NC, Priyanka DR, Madireddy N, Priyanka JN, Ramakrishna M, Ajay M, et al. Melasma Associated with Periodontitis, Anemia, and Vitamin D Abnormalities: A Chance Occurrence or a Syndrome. J Contemp Dent Pract. 2018;19:1254–9.

185. Abdalla DrM, Nayaf M, Hussein S. Evaluation of Vitamin D in Melasma Patients. Revista Romana de Medicina de Laborator. 2019;27:219–22.

186. P L. Worldwide Status of Vitamin D Nutrition [Internet]. The Journal of steroid biochemistry and molecular biology. J Steroid Biochem Mol Biol; 2010 [cited 2020 May 26]. Available from: https://pubmed.ncbi.nlm.nih.gov/20197091/

187. Jaishankar M, Tseten T, Anbalagan N, Mathew BB, Beeregowda KN. Toxicity, mechanism and health effects of some heavy metals. Interdiscip Toxicol. 2014;7:60–72.

188. Health C for D and R. Dental Amalgam Fillings [Internet]. FDA. FDA; 2021 [cited 2022 Apr 29]. Available from: https://www.fda.gov/medical-devices/dental-devices/dental-amalgam-fillings

189. Many products still contain mercury. These alternatives could replace them [Internet]. UNEP. 2019 [cited 2021 Nov 5]. Available from: http://www.unep.org/news-and-stories/story/many-products-still-contain-mercury-these-alternatives-could-replace-them

190. Anastasio M. Mercury spotlight: The toxic lamps that shall not be turned off [Internet]. META. 2019 [cited 2021 Oct 7]. Available from: https://meta.eeb.org/2019/12/05/mercury-spotlight-the-toxic-lamps-that-shall-not-be-turned-off/

191. Jagadeesan S, Duraisamy P, Panicker VV, Anjaneyan G, Sajini L, Velayudhan S, et al. Cutaneous mercury granulomas, hyperpigmentation and systemic involvement: A case of mercury toxicity following herbal medication for psoriasis. IJDVL. Scientific Scholar; 2021;87:892–892.

192. Nylander M, Weiner J. Relation between mercury and selenium in pituitary glands of dental staff. Br J Ind Med. 1989;46:751–2.

193. Møller-Madsen B, Thorlacius-Ussing O. Accumulation of mercury in the anterior pituitary of rats following oral or intraperitoneal administration of methyl mercury. Virchows Arch B Cell Pathol Incl Mol Pathol. 1986;51:303–11.

194. Danscher G, Hørsted-Bindslev P, Rungby J. Traces of mercury in organs from primates with amalgam fillings. Exp Mol Pathol. 1990;52:291–9.

195. Khayat A, Dencker L. Organ and cellular distribution of inhaled metallic mercury in the rat and Marmoset monkey (Callithrix jacchus): influence of ethyl alcohol pretreatment. Acta Pharmacol Toxicol (Copenh). 1984;55:145–52.

196. Lamperti AA, Printz RH. Localization, accumulation, and toxic effects of mercuric chloride on the reproductive axis of the female hamster. Biol Reprod. 1974;11:180–6.

197. Stadnicka A. Localization of mercury in the rat ovary after oral administration of mercuric chloride. Acta Histochem. 1980;67:227–33.

198. Nishida M, Yamamoto T, Yoshimura Y, Kawada J. Subacute toxicity of methylmercuric chloride and mercuric chloride on mouse thyroid. J Pharmacobiodyn. 1986;9:331–8.

199. Gerhard I, Runnebaum B. [The limits of hormone substitution in pollutant exposure and fertility disorders]. Zentralbl Gynakol. 1992;114:593–602.

200. Davis BJ, Price HC, O'Connor RW, Fernando R, Rowland AS, Morgan DL. Mercury vapor and female reproductive toxicity. Toxicol Sci. 2001;59:291–6.

201. Lamperti A, Niewenhuis R. The effects of mercury on the structure and function of the hypothalamo-pituitary axis in the hamster. Cell Tissue Res. 1976;170:315–24.

202. Rowland AS, Baird DD, Weinberg CR, Shore DL, Shy CM, Wilcox AJ. The effect of occupational exposure to mercury vapour on the fertility of female dental assistants. Occup Environ Med. 1994;51:28–34.

203. Solano F. On the Metal Cofactor in the Tyrosinase Family. Int J Mol Sci [Internet]. 2018 [cited 2020 Sep 22];19. Available from: https://www.ncbi.nlm.nih.gov/pmc/articles/PMC5855855/

204. Water NRC (US) C on C in D. Health Effects of Excess Copper [Internet]. Copper in Drinking Water. National Academies Press (US); 2000 [cited 2020 Sep 23]. Available from: https://www.ncbi. nlm.nih.gov/books/NBK225400/

205. Rani R, Sarin RC, Singh G. Serum Copper, Ceruloplasmin and Non Ceruloplasmin Copper Levels in Hyperpigmentary Disorders. Indian J Dermatol Venereol Leprol. 1978;44:134–7.

206. Tchounwou PB, Yedjou CG, Patlolla AK, Sutton DJ. Heavy Metals Toxicity and the Environment. EXS. 2012;101:133–64.

207. Judge S, Sydney CN. The relationship between copper, oestrogen & anxiety [Internet]. Sydney Naturopath & Nutritionist. 2018 [cited 2021 Mar 27]. Available from: https://stevenjudge.com.au/ are-you-copper-toxic-sydney-naturopath/

208. Jasim S, Tjälve H. Effects of sodium pyridinethione on the uptake and distribution of nickel, cadmium and zinc in pregnant and non-pregnant mice. Toxicology. 1986;38:327–50.

209. Lead Statistics and Information | U.S. Geological Survey [Internet]. [cited 2022 May 2]. Available from: https://www.usgs.gov/centers/national-minerals-information-centerlead-statistics -and-information

210. Toxic Chocolate — As You Sow [Internet]. [cited 2022 May 2]. Available from: https://www. asyousow.org/environmental-health/toxic-enforcement/toxic-chocolate

211. Outhman AM, Lamma OA. Investigate the contamination of tissue paper with heavy metals in the local market. International Journal of Chemical Studies. 2020;8:1264.

212. Pollack AZ, Schisterman EF, Goldman LR, Mumford SL, Albert PS, Jones RL, et al. Cadmium, Lead, and Mercury in Relation to Reproductive Hormones and Anovulation in Premenopausal Women. Environ Health Perspect. 2011;119:1156–61.

213. Dundar B, Oktem F, Arslan MK, Delibas N, Baykal B, Arslan C, et al. The effect of long-term low-dose lead exposure on thyroid function in adolescents. Environ Res. 2006;101:140–5.

214. Kasperczyk S, Birkner E, Kasperczyk A, Kasperczyk J. Lipids, lipid peroxidation and 7-ketocholesterol in workers exposed to lead. Hum Exp Toxicol. SAGE Publications Ltd STM; 2005;24:287–95.

215. factsheet22.pdf [Internet]. [cited 2022 Jan 29]. Available from: http://nmsp.cals.cornell.edu/ publications/factsheets/factsheet22.pdf

216. Too Much Sugar Turns Off Gene That Controls Effects Of Sex Steroids [Internet]. ScienceDaily. [cited 2022 Aug 19]. Available from: https://www.sciencedaily.com/releases/2007/11/071109171610. htm

217. Rice KM, Walker EM, Wu M, Gillette C, Blough ER. Environmental Mercury and Its Toxic Effects. J Prev Med Public Health. 2014;47:74–83.

218. Pinheiro MCN, Macchi BM, Vieira JLF, Oikawa T, Amoras WW, Guimarães GA, et al. Mercury exposure and antioxidant defenses in women: A comparative study in the Amazon. Environmental Research. 2008;107:53–9.

219. Jan AT, Azam M, Siddiqui K, Ali A, Choi I, Haq QMohdR. Heavy Metals and Human Health: Mechanistic Insight into Toxicity and Counter Defense System of Antioxidants. Int J Mol Sci.

2015;16:29592–630.

220. Jones MM. Heavy-Metal Detoxification Using Sulfur Compounds. Sulfur Reports [Internet]. Taylor & Francis Group; 2007 [cited 2022 May 7]; Available from: https://www.tandfonline.com/doi/abs/10.1080/01961778508082472

221. Abdulrazak S, Hussaini K, Sani HM. Evaluation of removal efficiency of heavy metals by low-cost activated carbon prepared from African palm fruit. Appl Water Sci. 2017;7:3151–5.

222. Saif MJ, Zia KM, Fazal-ur-Rehman null, Usman M, Hussain AI, Chatha SAS. Removal of Heavy Metals by Adsorption onto Activated Carbon Derived from Pine Cones of Pinus roxburghii. Water Environ Res. 2015;87:291–7.

223. Charcoal Detox Protocol [Internet]. Charcoal Times Blog. [cited 2022 May 8]. Available from: https://charcoaltimes.com/2694-2/

224. Thomas DD. Breathing new life into nitric oxide signaling: A brief overview of the interplay between oxygen and nitric oxide. Redox Biology. 2015;5:225–33.

225. Bernardi L, Passino C, Wilmerding V, Dallam GM, Parker DL, Robergs RA, et al. Breathing patterns and cardiovascular autonomic modulation during hypoxia induced by simulated altitude. J Hypertens. 2001;19:947–58.

226. "Let food be thy medicine"–Hippocrates? | Dr Goodfood [Internet]. [cited 2021 Nov 3]. Available from: https://www.drgoodfood.org/en/news/let-food-be-thy-medicine-hippocrates

227. Mead MN. Benefits of Sunlight: A Bright Spot for Human Health. Environ Health Perspect. 2008;116:A160–7.

228. Memme JM, Erlich AT, Phukan G, Hood DA. Exercise and mitochondrial health. The Journal of Physiology. 2021;599:803–17.

229. Breath by James Nestor [Internet]. [cited 2021 Jul 26]. Available from: https://www.penguin.com.au/books/breath-9780241289129

230. Madkour MI, El-Serafi AT, Jahrami HA, Sherif NM, Hassan RE, Awadallah S, et al. Ramadan diurnal intermittent fasting modulates SOD2, TFAM, Nrf2, and sirtuins (SIRT1, SIRT3) gene expressions in subjects with overweight and obesity. Diabetes Research and Clinical Practice [Internet]. Elsevier; 2019 [cited 2022 May 14];155. Available from: https://www.diabetesresearchclinicalpractice.com/article/S0168-8227(19)30217-7/fulltext

231. Lettieri-Barbato D, Cannata SM, Casagrande V, Ciriolo MR, Aquilano K. Time-controlled fasting prevents aging-like mitochondrial changes induced by persistent dietary fat overload in skeletal muscle. PLOS ONE. Public Library of Science; 2018;13:e0195912.

232. Nasr MA, Dovbeshko GI, Bearne SL, El-Badri N, Matta CF. Heat Shock Proteins in the "Hot" Mitochondrion: Identity and Putative Roles. Bioessays. 2019;41:e1900055.

233. Hafen PS, Preece CN, Sorensen JR, Hancock CR, Hyldahl RD. Repeated exposure to heat stress induces mitochondrial adaptation in human skeletal muscle. Journal of Applied Physiology. American Physiological Society; 2018;125:1447–55.

234. Chung N, Park J, Lim K. The effects of exercise and cold exposure on mitochondrial biogenesis in skeletal muscle and white adipose tissue. J Exerc Nutrition Biochem. 2017;21:39–47.

235. Núñez-Álvarez C, Del Olmo-Aguado S, Merayo-Lloves J, Osborne NN. Near infra-red light attenuates corneal endothelial cell dysfunction in situ and in vitro. Exp Eye Res. 2017;161:106–15.

236. Del Olmo-Aguado S, Núñez-Álvarez C, Osborne NN. Red light of the visual spectrum attenuates cell death in culture and retinal ganglion cell death in situ. Acta Ophthalmol. 2016;94:e481-491.

237. Beauvoit B, Kitai T, Chance B. Contribution of the mitochondrial compartment to the optical properties of the rat liver: a theoretical and practical approach. Biophys J. 1994;67:2501–10.

238. Hamblin MR. Mechanisms and Mitochondrial Redox Signaling in Photobiomodulation. Photochem Photobiol. 2018;94:199–212.

239. Wesselink E, Koekkoek W a. C, Grefte S, Witkamp RF, van Zanten ARH. Feeding mitochondria: Potential role of nutritional components to improve critical illness convalescence. Clin Nutr. 2019;38:982–95.

240. Watanabe F, Yabuta Y, Bito T, Teng F. Vitamin B12-Containing Plant Food Sources for Vegetarians. Nutrients. 2014;6:1861–73.

241. 10 Foods High in Vitamin B for Plant-Based and Meat-Eaters Alike | livestrong [Internet]. LIVESTRONG.COM. [cited 2022 May 15]. Available from: https://www.livestrong.com/article/13764952-foods-high-in-vitamin-b/

242. 15 Healthy Foods That Are High in Vitamin C [Internet]. Verywell Fit. [cited 2022 May 15]. Available from: https://www.verywellfit.com/foods-high-in-vitamin-c-2507745

243. Office of Dietary Supplements – Vitamin E [Internet]. [cited 2022 May 15]. Available from: https://ods.od.nih.gov/factsheets/VitaminE-HealthProfessional/

244. Selenium Foods: Top 21 Foods High in Selenium [Internet]. Greatist. 2020 [cited 2022 May 15]. Available from: https://greatist.com/eat/selenium-foods

245. The 20 Best Plant-Based Sources of Zinc [Internet]. ThePlantWay.com. 2020 [cited 2022 May 15]. Available from: http://www.theplantway.com/zinc-plant-based-sources/

246. Office of Dietary Supplements – Zinc [Internet]. [cited 2022 May 15]. Available from: https://ods.od.nih.gov/factsheets/Zinc-HealthProfessional/

247. Zhao H, Wu H, He J, Zhuang J, Liu Z, Yang Y, et al. Frontal cortical mitochondrial dysfunction and mitochondria-related β-amyloid accumulation by chronic sleep restriction in mice. Neuroreport. 2016;27:916–22.

248. Lu Z, Hu Y, Wang Y, Zhang T, Long J, Liu J. Topological reorganizations of mitochondria isolated from rat brain after 72 hours of paradoxical sleep deprivation, revealed by electron cryo-tomography. American Journal of Physiology-Cell Physiology. American Physiological Society; 2021;321:C17–25.

249. Huang W-H, Lee A-R, Yang C-H. Antioxidative and anti-inflammatory activities of polyhydroxyflavonoids of Scutellaria baicalensis GEORGI. Biosci Biotechnol Biochem. 2006;70:2371–80.

250. Kimura Y, Sumiyoshi M. Effects of various flavonoids isolated from Scutellaria baicalensis roots on skin damage in acute UVB-irradiated hairless mice. J Pharm Pharmacol. 2011;63:1613–23.

251. Joseph S. Sound Healing using Solfeggio Frequencies. 2019.

252. Akimoto K, Hu A, Yamaguchi T, Kobayashi H. Effect of 528 Hz Music on the Endocrine System and Autonomic Nervous System. Health. Scientific Research Publishing; 2018;10:1159–70.

253. Chevalier G, Sinatra ST, Oschman JL, Sokal K, Sokal P. Earthing: Health Implications of Reconnecting the Human Body to the Earth's Surface Electrons. Journal of Environmental and Public Health. Hindawi; 2012;2012:e291541.

254. Chevalier G. Grounding the Human Body Improves Facial Blood Flow Regulation: Results of a Randomized, Placebo Controlled Pilot Study. Journal of Cosmetics, Dermatological Sciences and Applications. Scientific Research Publishing; 2014;4:293–308.

255. Corn-Free Diet – Pediatric Nutrition – Golisano Children's Hospital – University of Rochester Medical Center [Internet]. [cited 2022 May 15]. Available from: https://www.urmc.rochester.edu/childrens-hospital/nutrition/corn-free.aspx

256. Sources of Gluten [Internet]. Celiac Disease Foundation. [cited 2022 May 15]. Available from:

https://celiac.org/gluten-free-living/what-is-gluten/sources-of-gluten/

257. Soy-Allergy-Avoidance-List-Hidden-Names.pdf [Internet]. [cited 2022 May 15]. Available from: https://www.kidswithfoodallergies.org/media/Soy-Allergy-Avoidance-List-Hidden-Names.pdf

258. 56 Different Names for Sugar in Your Food [Internet]. Verywell Fit. [cited 2022 Nov 8]. Available from: https://www.verywellfit.com/different-names-for-sugar-2242526

APPENDIX

QUESTIONNAIRE

When you answer the questions, please do not judge yourself and be kind to yourself. This is a roadmap to better skin and to find out where you are in your health journey. Please use the page on 182 for any additional notes.

GENERAL

When did melasma come up? Year.

Please do a quick brainstorm. What happened in that year (a stressful job, loss, separation, juggling family and work, illness or any other emotional hardship)?

Have you given birth or breastfed in the past or currently? If yes, was the onset of melasma around that time?

Are you currently experiencing stress emotionally or mentally?

Where did you live at onset of melasma (country, city)?

Where do you live at the moment?

What is your current work (homemaker and mother count)?

Do you have any health challenges?

Do you have allergies?

PART II IMBALANCES

Nervous system

Do you experience frequent headaches? If yes, how often? Where on the head are they usually located?

Are you a nose breather? Do you find yourself breathing fast and shallow or not breathing at times?

Endocrine System

Stress and Adrenals

Out of a scale from 1–10, 1 very little and 10 a lot. How would you rate the impact melasma has on your well-being? How does it impact your daily life?

Do you feel exhausted and fatigued and have low energy levels?

Have you had exposure to harsh chemicals on your skin (where melasma lesions are)?

Have you had injuries or any ablative (exfoliating) treatments on your skin (where melasma lesions are)?

Let us do some face reading. Do you have nasolabial folds that extend towards the chin? Do you have lines at the inner corner of the eye? Do you have dark circles?

If you have answered any of these questions with yes, it is likely that your stress load is too high or that your skin has experienced too much stress, which can cause or contribute to hyperpigmentation.

How do you cope with stress? Do you have tools/methods to reduce stress?

Thyroid

Do you have a thyroid condition you know of?

Do you feel anxious regularly?

Do you usually feel hot or cold?

Do you feel restless?

Have you had sudden weight gain or weight loss?

Are your skin, nails or hair dry or brittle?

If you have answered any of these questions with yes, it is possible that you have an imbalance. Getting thyroid levels tested could be a good step forward.

Which levels should be tested?

TPO, FT4, TSH, AbTG, TPO (these levels deviated from normal levels in melasma)

Estrogen

Have you used the contraceptive pill in the past or currently? If yes, has the melasma come up during that time?

Have you had any other hormone treatments e.g., for cancer? If yes, has the melasma come up during that time?

Have you ever had a copper IUD or currently have one?

Do you have mood swings?

Do you have a low libido?

Do you get hot flushes?

Do you suffer from sleep problems? If yes, please describe.

Do you do shift work?

Are you exposed to blue light daily for several hours (computer screen, bright artificial, fluorescent light)?

Do you drink alcohol regularly?

The factors above are active contributors to estrogen imbalances. If any of these apply to you, there might be a correlation to your melasma.

Do you receive daily sunlight? Especially the first and last hour before sunrise/ sunset.

Receiving sunlight at sunrise and sunset is a big help to regulate your hormone levels.

If you have a period:

Are your cycles irregular (regular means between 28–32 days)?

Are your periods painful (to the extent that you have to rely on painkillers)?

Do you have PMS symptoms?

Do you have sore breasts before your period?

If you have answered the questions with yes, you may have increased estrogen levels.

Immune System

Has your skin (at the melasma site) experienced damage from an external factor (physical injury, chemicals, excess heat or sun) shortly before the development of melasma?

Have you had a reaction to a cosmetic product shortly before melasma came up?

Do you have food sensitivities or a chronic gut condition? If yes, what kind?

Do you have digestive problems?

Oxidative Stress and Mitochondrial Health

Do you exercise regularly?

Do you wear blue blockers?

Do you work in an area with bright artificial lighting?

PART III FACTORS

Emotional stress

Do you feel like you have a high workload?

Do you feel overwhelmed with your daily tasks?

Endocrine Disruptors

Do you frequently drink from plastic bottles or eat from plastic containers?

Do you frequently use aluminium foil?

Is there a possible load of chemicals in your cooking ware e.g., non-stick pans, Teflon?

Is there a possible load of chemicals in your carpets, clothing, and other textiles?

Do you use organic and clean cosmetic products?

Do you use deodorant with aluminium?

Do you use natural/non-toxic cleaning products including washing detergent?

Mold

Do you live in a water damaged house or have you been exposed mold somewhere else?

Do you have allergy symptoms (runny nose, itchy and red eyes, sneezing, coughing)?

Are you sensitive to certain chemicals but not allergic?

Do you have brain fog?

Do you often feel depressed?

Do you sense a metallic taste in your mouth?

Medication

Are you taking any medication at the moment?

Have you taken any of the following medications: chloroquine, chlorpromazine, clomipramine?

Have you had long term use of antibiotics?

Diet

Do you have a nutrient-dense diet?

What percentage of your food is organic?

How many times do you eat takeaway or ready-to-eat meals weekly?

Are you taking any supplements?

Gut Microbiome

Are you taking any probiotics at the moment or in the past?

Have you taken probiotics after a course of antibiotics?

Do you have any other skin conditions other than melasma?

Heat, Chemicals in Cosmetics and Physical Stressors

Are you using any cosmetic products with the following ingredients?

- Essential oils (phototoxicity)

- Alcohol (Ethanol)

- Perfume/fragrance

- AHA/BHA

Have you had the following treatments on your face?

- Laser

- Peels

- Skin needling

- Other facials

- Light treatments

Have you had any other advanced skin treatments?

Air Pollution and Hypoxia

Are you frequently exposed to exhaust, e.g. at work?

Do you know your iron levels (oxygenation of cells is vital to skin health)?

Artificial Light, UV and Vit D

Do you sit by the window at work?

Do you drive daily at peak sun hours (between 10 am and 4 pm)?

Do you know your vitamin D levels?

Do you get sunshine daily?

Are you wearing sunscreen during peak hours?

Do you work outdoors during peak hours?

Metals

Mercury

Do you have amalgam fillings?

Copper

Do you drink water from the tap? (Look for green or blue residue around faucets in the house. If that is the case, copper is likely to be high in your tap water.)

Nickel

Do you wear fake jewellery?

Lead

Does the wall paint in your house or furniture contain lead?

Lead tests are available in hardware stores. If your wall paint or interior has lead and the paint is chipping or cracking, you might have lead exposure.

Those questions can help you to explore your own melasma story and narrow down the root cause for you.

For an evaluation of your questionnaire and a customised protocol, you can send me a photograph of your answers to: janett@ecvilibria.com (fees apply).

Please visit ecvilibria.com for more information.

NOTES

TABLE OF INFLAMMATORY FOODS AND FOOD ADDITIVES

MOST INFLAMMATORY FOODS AND FOOD ADDITIVES TO AVOID:				
CORN	**WHEAT**	**SOY**	**SUGAR**	**FATS**
Corn flour	Wheat varieties and derivatives of wheat such as:	Soy flour	Fructose	Omega 6 (if not well balanced with Omega 3)
Cornmeal		Soybean flour	Sucrose	
Corn gluten		Soy lecithin	Barley malt syrup	
Cornflakes	Wheatberries	Bean curd		Trans fats from:
Corn starch (listed on labels as starch or vegetable starch)	Durum	Edamame	Beet sugar	Vegetable oils
	Emmer	Soybeans	Blackstrap molasses	Margarines
	Semolina	Soy formula		
Corn oil	Spelt	Soy milk	Brown rice syrup	
Corn syrup	Farina	Soybean paste	Brown sugar	
High fructose corn syrup	Farro	Hydrolysed soy protein	Buttered syrup	
	Graham		Cane crystals (or cane juice crystals)	
Dextrin	KAMUT®	Soy grits		
Maltodextrins	Khorasan wheat	Supro	Cane sugar	
Dextrose	Einkorn wheat	Kinnoko flour	Caramel	
Fructose		Soy miso	Carob syrup	
Crystalline fructose	Rye	Tamari	Castor sugar	
	Barley	Kyodofu	Confectioner's sugar (powdered sugar)	
Treacle	Triticale	Soy nuts		
Ethanol		Soy nut butter		
Free fatty acids		Tempeh	Corn sweetener	
Maize		Miso	Corn syrup	
		Soy protein		

MOST INFLAMMATORY FOODS AND FOOD ADDITIVES TO AVOID (CONTINUED):

CORN	WHEAT	SOY	SUGAR	FATS
Zein	Malt in various forms including:	Teriyaki sauce	Corn syrup solids	
Sorbitol [255]		Natto concentrate	Date sugar	
MSG (Monosodium glutamate is a flavour enhancer that can be derived from corn, wheat and sugars)	Malted barley flour	Soy protein	Demerara sugar	
	Malted milk or milkshakes	Textured soy flour	Dehydrated cane juice	
	Malt extract	Okara isolate	Dextrin	
	Malt syrup	Textured soy protein	Dextrose	
	Malt flavouring	Shoyu sauce	Evaporated cane juice	
	Malt vinegar	Soy sauce	Florida crystals	
	Brewer's Yeast	Soy albumin	Fruit juice	
	Wheat Starch	Soy sprouts	Fruit juice concentrate	
	MSG (Monosodium glutamate) [256]	Tofu	Glucose	
		Soy bran	Golden sugar	
		Soy fibre	Golden syrup	
		Soya	Grape sugar	
		Soya flour	Icing sugar	
		Yakidofu	Invert sugar	
		Soy concentrate	Lactose	
		Soybean granules	Maltodextrin	
		Yuba	Malt syrup	
		Soybean curd [257]	Maltose	
			Molasses	
			Muscovado sugar	
			Palm sugar	

MOST INFLAMMATORY FOODS AND FOOD ADDITIVES TO AVOID (CONTINUED):

CORN	WHEAT	SOY	SUGAR	FATS
			Panela sugar	
			Raw sugar	
			Refiner's syrup	
			Rice syrup	
			Saccharose	
			Sorghum syrup	
			Sucanat	
			Syrup	
			Treacle	
			Turbinado sugar	
			Yellow sugar	
			Xylose	
			[258]	
			(Ingredients ending	
			with -ose are sugars)	
			Alcohol	
			Artificial sweeteners	
			like:	
			Aspartame	
			MSG (Monosodium	
			glutamate)	

Table 13: Inflammatory foods and their derivatives.

INDEX

ABOUT THE AUTHOR

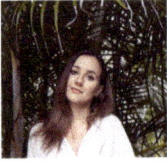

Janett is a cosmetic scientist and aesthetician. Her mission is to bring awareness surrounding the link between common skin concerns and our current environmental conditions to skin professionals and people affected by skin disorders. During the 17 years of her career as an aesthetician, she observed that specific skin conditions, such as melasma, are on the rise. Her work combines modern clinical research with a holistic, root cause-based treatment approach. She has managed her own chronic health and skin conditions by following the lifestyle approach she proposes in her work.

www.ingramcontent.com/pod-product-compliance
Lightning Source LLC
Chambersburg PA
CBHW041256040426
42334CB00028BA/3046